"It is one of the most beautiful compensations of life, that no man can sincerely try to help another without helping himself."
—Ralph Waldo Emerson

PRAISE FOR *ACHIEVE YOUR VICTORY*

Dr. Daniel Klauer has established himself as a leader among an expanding nucleus of collaborators from diverse fields of practice united by a common purpose: identifying and treating the airway and breathing problems that drive a host of health conditions. Careful reflection on patterns he recognized in his clinical practice and insights gained from conversations with others involved in the care of patients with airway problems piqued Dr. Klauer's curiosity about the possibility that many prevalent health issues might have a common precursor. Recognizing the impact this area of practice can have on a patient's health and well being, Dr. Klauer has sought to improve access to this specialized care by organizing conferences and symposia where other practitioners can hear case reports, review literature, and learn to apply new techniques in their efforts to improve their patients' lives. It has been a privilege to collaborate with Dr. Klauer and I look forward to our future endeavors.

Darius Loghmanee, MD
Pediatric Sleep Medicine

Dr. Klauer's sense of victory includes this notion that there is no victory unless everyone has tried their best to deliver and receive the proper care. A great outcome will be short-lived if either the professional or the patient do not invest their best efforts in caring and being cared for. The collaborative multi-professional approach Dr. Klauer outlines in this book is a testimony to the best practice of medicine where egos too big to admit new learning, turf battles, and non-compliant patients are alien concepts. The joy of health care is caring and being cared for, and if you allow this, then you will receive the most beautiful compensation of life where both sides experience victory.

Roger Klauer, MD, MDiv

Physical Medicine & Rehabilitation

To successfully treat patients with pain disorders, we must look beyond the obvious issue the patient is complaining of and be able to assess the entire patient, including mind, body and spirit. Dr. Daniel Klauer and I are kindred spirits in this respect. He and I have worked together for the past four years evaluating and treating challenging and acute, but mostly chronic pain patients. He and Dr. Steven Olmos have opened my eyes to the depth of sleep medicine and the influence of jaw disorders on the mechanics and function of the entire body, and they have given me new, physical examination skills to better assess my patients and achieve more consistent outcomes with precise, targeted treatment. In a time when we must stop symptomatically treating pain with narcotics and steroids, Dr. Klauer's skills bring a refreshing and critical approach to the management of head, neck and jaw pain disorders.

Mark Cantieri, DO

Author and owner of Corrective Care

Dr. Klauer has helped change my practice and provide better treatment for patients with sleep and temporomandibular joint issues. He provides a comprehensive approach that seeks to understand the underlying issues and develop the expertise to provide the correct treatment. In my role as a sports medicine physician, his ability to help athletes improve their function and performance has been quite significant. I trust him both with my patients and my own family.

Mat Leiszler, MD
Sports Medicine

Dr. Klauer has brought great insight to our community and I am grateful for that. He has challenged traditional teachings and helped educate clinicians in current evidence-based care. Finally, patients in this community are getting the care that they truly need. No longer are we simply treating the symptoms of our patients' pain and dysfunction. Today, we can diagnose and treat the root of their problem, getting lasting results—no more band aids. I have been impressed with the multidisciplinary approach to patient care and I am happy to have him as a resource for my patients. Dr. Klauer has established and educated a network of medical and dental professionals. Through this collaboration, all facets of patient care can be addressed. Thank you Dr. Klauer for putting together a concise resource for both our colleagues and our patients!

Dr. Chad Harrington, DDS, MS
Board-Certified Orthodontist and owner of Harrington Orthodontics

An extraordinary and compassionate dentist, Dr. Daniel Klauer has entered into a new paradigm of medicine: finding the true source of your pain—not merely treating your symptoms. He is determined to treat you naturally, without unnecessary surgery or medication.

If you want to relieve your pain and improve your sleep, you must read this book. Who would have thought that breathing and sleeping were so important? Dr. Klauer has taught me how to challenge the traditional way of practicing medicine. In his book, he will show you how all fields of medicine must work together to improve your health and improve your life.

I am a better physician because of Dr. Klauer. My health and my sleep are much improved, and yours can be too.

Victor Romano, MD

Romano Orthopaedics Center

As a sports medicine and sports performance team, we know the system Dr. Klauer has delivered to our athletes has prevented injuries, improved treatment, and enhanced performance. His evaluation, assessment, guidance, and creation of a plan of care for our athletes addresses the root cause of a specific condition. This has allowed us to better serve our patients and improve outcomes.

Rob Hunt, EdM, ATC

Director of Athletic Training and Rehabilitative Services

With the publication of this book, Dr. Klauer has given health-care providers, and the recipients of the care that they provide, a precious resource. Within these pages, the reader will become scientifically enlightened about how several of the chronic health problems that are so highly prevalent in today's industrialized societies are not only treatable without drugs or invasive surgeries, but also mostly preventable if specific environmental "triggers" are eliminated at their earliest recognition—in adults, and especially early childhood. For instance, over a few paragraphs subtitled "Sean's Victory," Dr. Klauer eloquently describes, in detail, how he rescued a five year-old child who had been referred to him per recurrent obstructive sleep apnea symptoms despite having previously had his tonsils and adenoids surgically removed. I would recommend this book to any healthcare provider who is involved in the sleep and respiratory wellness care of children and/or their adult caregivers; I also highly recommend it to those adult caregivers as the writing style is not overly "medical," but clear, entertaining, and most importantly, scientifically supported.

Thank you Dr.Klauer for this valuable gift!

Kevin L. Boyd, DDS, MSc

Pediatric Dentist and owner of Dentistry for Children and Families

ACHIEVE YOUR VICTORY

DR. DANIEL KLAUER

ACHIEVE YOUR
VICTORY

SOLUTIONS FOR

TMD AND SLEEP APNEA

Advantage®

Published by Advantage, Charleston, South Carolina.
Member of Advantage Media Group.

ADVANTAGE is a registered trademark, and the Advantage colophon is a trademark of Advantage Media Group, Inc.

10 9 8 7 6 5 4 3 2 1

ISBN: 978-1-59932-903-1
LCCN: 2018951133

Cover design by Carly Blake.
Layout design by Megan Elger.

This publication is designed to provide accurate and authoritative information in regard to the subject matter covered. It is sold with the understanding that the publisher is not engaged in rendering legal, accounting, or other professional services. If legal advice or other expert assistance is required, the services of a competent professional person should be sought.

Advantage Media Group is proud to be a part of the Tree Neutral® program. Tree Neutral offsets the number of trees consumed in the production and printing of this book by taking proactive steps such as planting trees in direct proportion to the number of trees used to print books. To learn more about Tree Neutral, please visit **www. treeneutral.com.**

Advantage Media Group is a publisher of business, self-improvement, and professional development books and online learning. We help entrepreneurs, business leaders, and professionals share their Stories, Passion, and Knowledge to help others Learn & Grow. Do you have a manuscript or book idea that you would like us to consider for publishing? Please visit **advantagefamily.com** or call **1.866.775.1696.**

To Hayley, my loving wife, and our children,
Carson, Maddie, Nicholas, and Lena.

TABLE OF CONTENTS

ACKNOWLEDGMENTS

Thank you, Hayley, for loving me, supporting me, and always encouraging me to be better … I love you!

Thank you, Mom, for being the best example of unconditional, selfless, endless love and compassion. You are truly amazing and one of a kind.

Thank you, Dad, for showing me that as a provider, you can dramatically impact a patient's life even beyond their chief complaint. Thank you for keeping me grounded and humble, and for showing me how to love God, my wife, and family first.

Thank you, Uncle Rocky, for giving me the confidence and encouragement to speak toe-to-toe with physicians of all specialties.

Thank you, Papa Klauer, for quietly encouraging me and praying for my success. Although you somehow always knew my career path, you let me find my way.

Thank you, Dr. Mahoney, for introducing me to the profession of dentistry and welcoming me into your practice.

Thank you, Dr. Olmos, for putting together the most comprehensive clinical protocols to literally transform patients' lives. Thank you for accepting me as your student and pioneering the way in this field of medicine and dentistry.

Thank you, Scott Manning, for being such a great friend and leader, and ensuring I achieve the goals for my family, my practice, and my life. You are truly one of a kind.

ABOUT THE AUTHOR

A lifelong resident of Granger, Indiana, Daniel Klauer, DDS, has strong ties to his Midwest community. He attended the University of Notre Dame and was a member of the Big East Championship Varsity Golf Team. After graduating from the University of Notre Dame, Dr. Klauer earned his doctor of dental surgery degree (DDS) from The Ohio State University.

Since 2013, after seeing an overwhelming need, Dr. Klauer chose to limit his practice to treating patients with craniofacial pain, TMD (temporomandibular joint disorders), and sleep breathing disorders. As he learned to identify the origin of patients' pain and sleep problems, it became increasingly clear that he could drastically impact their lives now and in the future.

Dr. Klauer is board-certified with the American Board of Dental Sleep Medicine, American Board of Craniofacial Pain, and the American Board of Craniofacial Dental Sleep Medicine. He is diplomate eligible with the American Board of Orofacial Pain and currently is the only doctor in a hundred-mile radius of South Bend, Indiana who carries these three board credentials.

Dr. Klauer enjoys educating patients and giving them the tools to live healthier lives independent of medications and quick fixes. He has a compassion for patients that is evident in the welcoming environment of his practice, his dedication to ongoing learning, and his commitment to improving the industry by sharing his knowledge with colleagues as a lecturer around the world.

Dr. Klauer also works with the University of Notre Dame Athletic Department, helping athletes be their best in the game. He proudly has been a part of screening athletes for sleep disordered breathing as well as treating several of the athletes with chronic headaches and other chronic ailments. By invitation, he has helped them implement Motor Nerve Reflex Testing (to be discussed in the book) as a screening tool for player performance, balance assessment, and injury prevention. Being a former student athlete at Notre Dame, this has been a fun way to give back to the University he has strong ties to.

Outside the office, Dr. Klauer enjoys life with his wife, Hayley, and his four young children. Together, they enjoy almost any outdoor activity, especially running, biking, and skiing.

FOREWORD

BY DR. DOUGLAS LIEPERT, MD

I believe a primary weakness in patient care revolves around each specialty focusing on what they can deliver with no collaboration. We have to understand each other's role and treatment options, or the patient will be doomed to hear only what we offer individually. I want to work with colleagues who focus on the diagnosis first and then figure out how to best treat the patient. This is what I receive from Dr. Klauer. I had met many dentists before I was introduced to Dr Klauer, but it was immediately clear he would be a great colleague. His dad is an MD, so he understood diagnosis, and his interest lay in treating the patient, not in delivery of an appliance or doing a procedure.

I was introduced to Dr. Klauer by chance after he started his journey in dental sleep medicine and TMD treatment. He had asked my facial plastics partner if he knew any ENTs interested in sleep. My partner's reply was that it just so happens we just hired a partner board-certified in sleep. I have always focused on a comprehensive and multidisciplinary path towards caring for patients with sleep disorders. I preached the philosophy that sleep was as diverse as cancer and required a multi-specialist approach. Dr. Klauer is a key member of my circle of care because he shares this philosophy, and this sets him apart from the weekend warriors who have just enough knowledge to focus on the oral appliance. His evaluations are comprehensive and focused on identifying all of his patients' diagnosis. He is also very skilled with the treatment of craniofacial pain. This often needs no MD collaboration, but when he also identifies a sleep component, he does not hesitate to consult. It is not that he does not understand sleep. With all his training and four years of our collaboration, he just understands the power of the team. I have not once seen him deliver a sleep appliance until we had completed this process. We work as colleagues in the same manner as I do with my neurology and pulmonologist sleep physicians. He is truly a doctor of dental sleep medicine.

I have watched his practice grow as he incorporated new treatments and diagnostic tools, recognizing his patients' needs. It was an honor to be his sponsor as he moved through the process of the dental sleep boards. We had many fun nights looking at polysomnograms and meeting together to develop individual care plans for patients. Rarely did patients have only a single sleep or pain problem. Over the last four years, it has become clear that it does not really matter who the patient sees first. We would help the patient get what they needed. It did not matter whether it was surgery, an OA, myofunctional therapy, or CPAP. We have taught each other how to be a unique team which we hope will change the paradigm from the silo of the sleep lab to a multispecialty team helping people with sleep and pain disorders.

Douglas R. Liepert, MD
Board-Certified in ENT & Sleep Medicine
Michiana Sleep Solutions
Allied ENT Specialty Center
Research Professor University of Notre Dame

FOREWORD

BY DR. STEVEN OLMOS, DDS

I have dedicated my life to helping people with chronic pain and breathing disorders. Having focused my almost forty years of practice in this effort, and I have produced and taught continuing education courses around the world to share my treatment paradigms with physicians, dentists and other health care providers. I met Dr. Daniel Klauer when he attended these courses. It is an understatement to say he is an exceptional student who understands the importance of a road-tested system to achieve treatment success and is able to implement them.

Through my years of teaching, I have come to realize there are a handful of students that have the gift of comprehension, assimilation, conversion, and most importantly, the ability to make complicated things simple. In reading this book, it's clear that Dr. Daniel Klauer is one of these special handfuls. Humility is the gift of greatness.

He explains concepts in this book clearly so that anyone can understand them without a background of knowledge. He explains these concepts with cases that demonstrate conditions that are likely familiar to someone you love or know. It is possible that you are deciding to read this book because you suffer from these ailments. If so, you have made the right choice to pick it up, and I am sure you will find direction for relief of your symptoms.

People, such as Dr. Daniel Klauer, who focus on helping others with chronic pain and breathing dysfunction, are a special breed. They are fueled by the relief of suffering by others and the improved quality of life. It is what we all strive for. Feeling good and healthy without the assistance of medications that give an illusion of health.

I am proud of all my students and the Centre concept that standardizes these protocols. This book makes me especially proud.

Well done Dr. Klauer.

Steven R. Olmos, DDS, DABCP, DABCDSM, DAAPM, DABDSM, FAAOP, FAACP, FICCMO, FADI, FIAO
Founder, TMJ & Sleep Therapy Centres International

INTRODUCTION
A JOURNEY TO WELLNESS

If you have a rock in your right shoe, your right foot will hurt. But it's also likely that your *left* knee and hip will start hurting, because unconsciously, you keep taking pressure off your right foot so that you won't feel that rock jabbing you all the time. Eventually, you'll forget about the rock because the pain in your knee and hip are so bad. If you go to a doctor who only examines your left knee and hip where you're reporting pain, he or she might suggest treatment or have no answers, when all that's really needed is for a doctor to look in your right shoe and remove the rock. That's because in chronic pain situations, the chief complaint is rarely the origin of the problem.

The term "allopathic medicine" was coined in 1810 by Samuel Hahnemann. In doctor-speak, allopathic medicine is defined as "pharmacologically active agents or physical interventions to treat or suppress symptoms of pathophysiologic processes of diseases." In simpler terms, it is Western medicine, the modern medicine system in use today. Allopathic medicine, by definition, dictates that providers look at what the patient says is the problem—the symptom. But medicine is hopefully heading in a new direction, involving looking at the patient from head to toe to figure out the "why" to find the source of the problem. This new direction is nothing new, but rather the way the practice of medicine originally took flight—treating the source of the problem, not just masking the symptoms. It is important to identify the cause of a problem before doctors start treatment.

Although I am a doctor of dental surgery (DDS), my job today is to "look in the right shoe" to get to the source of patients' chronic facial pain and sleep problems. I look for the cause of a problem before I start treatment. In that regard, and others, I'm in a unique position to answer questions that other providers may not be able to answer. That's how my patients get relief and a second chance at better health.

The way I practice today is an evolution from where I began. Like most dentists, I used to fill cavities, crown teeth, perform root canals, extract teeth, and so on. I really enjoyed the work, but I felt there was a missing piece of the puzzle.

When I was in dental school, I always had questions about why people had broken teeth, jaw pain, and other problems. In fact, in 2005, for my medical physics class as an undergraduate at the University of Notre Dame, I did a research project on the nociceptive trigeminal inhibition reflex (this is the reflex that causes you to stop biting or open abruptly when you bite down too hard on a nut or hard substance when chewing), which is associated with the treatment of sleep-related bruxism, or what is commonly referred to as the clenching and grinding of teeth. But at that point in dental school, we were taught to create mouth guards for such problems, which treated the symptoms but not the root cause. It was a little like filling a cavity without educating the patient about the importance of keeping teeth clean—the reason they had the cavity in the first place. I was seeing patients who were sick but didn't even know that I could help them.

Then I went to a continuing education course that discussed craniofacial pain and sleep apnea, and suddenly everything clicked. As my mentor, and now great friend Dr. Steven Olmos says often, "It was like a bomb went off."

I came from a family of medical professionals: my great grandfather was a physician, my grandfather is a dentist, my dad is a physician, one uncle and my brother-in-law are dentists, and there are five nurses and five orthopedic surgeons in the family. So I always felt I was destined to care for patients in some manner.

Still, as of my junior year in college, I had not yet decided on a particular path. Then one day, while having my teeth cleaned by my family dentist, Dr. Terrance Mahoney at Mahoney Family Dentistry, I was invited to shadow him. That's when I really connected with my passion and I became motivated to make dentistry my career. It was through shadowing Dr. Mahoney that allowed me to connect with my Papa Klauer (a dentist) on a professional level. Little did I know but Papa Klauer was pioneering this field of dentistry and I didn't even begin to know the half of it.

When I was an undergraduate at the University of Notre Dame, my father gave me some great advice: "Identify a mentor to have in your career, because you will need them to progress as a professional." My father did his medical residencies (internal medicine and physical medicine and rehabilitation) at the Mayo Clinic in Rochester, Minnesota, for six years, where he was given a mentor to follow, emulate, and use throughout his residency. That was an essential piece in his medical training, and he always held it in high regard. And since I—and his patients—have always held him in high regard, I have studiously followed his advice, which in this case is quite tasking and time consuming, as I have four other mentors in my life.

After graduating from Ohio State University College of Dentistry in 2010, I began practicing with Dr. Mahoney. In 2012, the practice purchased a 3-D x-ray imaging device known as an i-CAT, and that same year, I learned about Dr. Olmos. Through his courses, I learned how to treat patients who have craniofacial pain, temporomandibular disorders (TMD), headaches, sleep apnea, snoring, and breathing issues. It was three years of intense training that involved traveling internationally, spending time at each other's offices, and many hours of private mentoring. I vividly remember discussing the anticipated journey with my wife, Hayley, since it required countless nights away from home. It was a whirlwind journey, but it was absolutely essential for putting me on the cutting edge in a specialty that crosses over into a new area of medicine. I am forever grateful for Dr. Olmos's tutelage, which has been so instrumental in my career, and for him sharing that experience in the foreword to this book.

As I began treating patients for pain, TMD, and sleep breathing disorders (SBD), it almost became an addiction to treat more and more of the same. After years of seeing patients who were dealing with chronic pain, lack of sleep, and other medical problems, the solutions we were implementing were helping people feel better almost immediately in many cases.

In regard to this notion of TMD and TMJ, I'd like to make a clarification. TMJ refers to the temporomandibular joints, which are located on each side of the face. Everyone has TMJ—in fact, we all have two TMJs, a left one and a right one. When patients say, "I have TMJ," what they truly mean is that they have a *disorder* or *dysfunction* of the TMJ. To avoid confusion, I often use the term "TM joint" when I'm talking about the anatomical structure of the temporomandibular joint versus TMD, the disorder that affects the joint.

So we evolved the practice to total wellness, an approach that takes a whole-body perspective to health rather than compartmentalizing medical issues within individual body systems. Today I focus mainly on issues in the mouth, jaw, and face, with the understanding that issues in these parts of the body may be generated within those structures or may be brought on by pain or misalignment in other parts of the body. Problems in the head, neck, or mouth negatively affect breathing and sleep, which then leads to additional health problems. Since everything in the body is connected, I look not only deeper within my own area of practice but also at the interrelationships between my specialty and other areas of medicine. This new approach is putting us at the forefront of what is going to be a mainstay in medicine and dentistry; it is simply a matter of time.

Today, my mission is to give hope to every person out there who is suffering from craniofacial pain, TMD, headaches, poor sleep, or problems they simply can't solve. My practice's mission statement is:

At the TMJ & Sleep Therapy Centre of Northern Indiana, we are committed to giving hope to patients of all ages by adopting their personal victory as our own. We restore the quality of life they deserve by providing the tools and therapies to decrease pain, increase energy, and improve sleep.

Our core values are:

- To embody integrity and authenticity in our relationships with patients and with each other. We empower all who enter our practice to be the best versions of themselves physically, emotionally, and spiritually.

- A commitment to lifelong learning, professionally and personally, to create an environment that breeds greatness. Obstacles are viewed as opportunities for improvement.

- To offer hope to patients by addressing the origin of their problems and focusing on their overall health and wellness.

- To be passionate about our purpose. Our passion unites us as a team to better understand our purpose and show compassion and empathy to our patients.

- To build relationships with transparent communication. At the first point of contact, we initiate the responsibility to create an honest, personable relationship with each patient through transparent communication. We don't impose our assumptions, we let our patients lead us to why they are seeking treatment.

It's a great feeling to be able to give people their lives back, and that's why I put this book together. I want patients to be able to make informed decisions about their health, and my goal is to begin that education before people even walk through the doors of my practice. The more that people know up front, the faster they can get better and the healthier they can be.

The cases in the chapters ahead are true stories, although the names are modified to protect privacy. These are recent stories among the thousands of patients we have been able to help. We welcome about seventy-five new patients a month, so choosing a handful was challenging, but I tried to share a variety of countless success stories.

This book is for people who are suffering from jaw pain stemming from TMD, craniofacial pain, headaches, snoring, SBD, and/or sleep apnea.[1] These dysfunctions will be explained in greater detail in the chapters ahead.

There are some common symptoms that may indicate a problem with a TMD or SBD. Look over these lists and mark those that you or a loved one is experiencing. Don't try to justify them, just simply mark "yes" or "no." I will refer to these lists in the chapters ahead.

---

1   When I refer to the jaw or jaws, I am talking about the upper jaw, the maxilla, and the lower jaw, the mandible. Moving forward, I will simply use the terms maxilla and mandible when referring to the upper and lower jaw.

PAIN OR TMD SYMPTOMS

- ☐ Headache pain
- ☐ Ear pain
- ☐ Jaw pain
- ☐ Chewing pain
- ☐ Face pain
- ☐ Eye pain
- ☐ Throat pain
- ☐ Neck pain
- ☐ Shoulder pain
- ☐ Back pain
- ☐ Limited ability to open mouth
- ☐ Difficulty closing mouth
- ☐ Jaw joint locking
- ☐ Jaw joint noises
- ☐ Stuffiness
- ☐ Sinus congestion
- ☐ Dizziness
- ☐ Ringing in the ears
- ☐ Muscle spasms
- ☐ Vision problems
- ☐ Numbness
- ☐ Nerve pain

SBD SYMPTOMS

- ☐ Acid indigestion
- ☐ Kicking or jerking leg repeatedly
- ☐ Swelling in ankles or feet
- ☐ Morning hoarseness in voice
- ☐ Dry mouth upon waking
- ☐ Fatigue
- ☐ Difficulty falling asleep
- ☐ Frequent tossing and turning
- ☐ Repeated awakening
- ☐ Nighttime urination
- ☐ Significant daytime drowsiness
- ☐ Frequent heavy snoring
- ☐ Feeling unrefreshed in the morning
- ☐ Affecting sleep of others
- ☐ Gasping upon waking
- ☐ Told that "I stop breathing" during sleep
- ☐ Nighttime choking spells
- ☐ Morning headaches
- ☐ Night sweats
- ☐ Vivid dreaming
- ☐ Unable to tolerate CPAP
- ☐ Teeth grinding
- ☐ Teeth crowding

My father always told me that as a doctor, I can only care for my patients as much as they are willing to care for themselves. That doesn't mean I should not give my patients everything I have in the way of knowledge and expertise about their issue, but that I should not take it personally if they fail to comply with my recommendations and guidance.

THE MORE YOU KNOW

My goal is to educate, motivate, and help my patients through their journey to wellness. The more you know, and the more you are willing to make the necessary changes, the better your chances are of having a great outcome from treatment. With you "at the table," we can address your symptoms and persevere in finding a way to help you enjoy the highest level of health throughout your life.

Investing in this book is a great first step, because the more you understand your condition and options, the more we can improve your outcomes.

In the pages ahead, you'll read about what my team and I call "victories." These are the ideal outcomes that each patient would like to achieve with treatment through our office.

For now, consider the answers to these questions.

WHY ARE YOU READING THIS BOOK?

_____

_____

_____

_____

WHAT WOULD BE A VICTORY
FOR YOU TODAY?

_____

_____

_____

_____

_____

Bring these answers to your consultation with me and my team at the TMJ & Sleep Therapy Centre of Northern Indiana. If you forget them, don't worry; my team gathers this information at every new patient appointment. Why? That's how we gauge our success, by how well we helped you achieve your victory. Read on to learn more about how we can help you do just that.

CHAPTER 1
ENVISION YOUR VICTORY

Discipline is the bridge between
goals and accomplishment.
—Jim Rohn

Whenever patients come for their first appointment at the TMJ & Sleep Therapy Centre of Northern Indiana, one of the first things we explore is the top three health concerns they want resolved—and winning over those problems is what's known as their "victory." Victories are the ideal outcomes patients want from treatment. For fifty-one-year-old Mary, those three problems, in her words, were heavy snoring, migraine headaches, and trouble falling asleep. But Mary wasn't ready to stop there—she was also chronically fatigued and frequently awoke with a dry mouth and extremely stiff shoulders, so those were added to the "victories" her treatment would target.

Mary had already been diagnosed with obstructive sleep apnea (OSA) by a board-certified sleep physician, who recommended for treatment either a continuous positive airway pressure (CPAP) machine (I'll go into more detail about this in Chapter 8) or an oral appliance, which is a specific and customized mouthpiece that aids with obstructive breathing at night. If those two options were ineffective, then surgery would be considered. While CPAP is a very effective treatment, it comes with a number of drawbacks that may keep patients from using it regularly, so Mary elected to first try an oral appliance. That led her to my practice.

—— VICTORY ——

For fifty-one-year-old Mary, those three problems, in her words, were heavy snoring, migraine headaches, and trouble falling asleep.
But Mary wasn't ready to stop there—she was also chronically fatigued and frequently awoke with a dry mouth and extremely stiff shoulders, so those were added to the "victories" her treatment would target.

When I refer to specialists, assume they are "board-certified" —doctors that have extensive time, training, and a certification examination process that solidifies their authority in that field.

In reviewing Mary's medical history during her first visit, a number of other issues surfaced. She had high blood pressure, an under-producing thyroid, anxiety, chronic fatigue, poor circulation, chronic sinus problems, and memory lapses—and she had recently gained quite a bit of weight. During her pregnancies, she had suffered from preeclampsia, which is high blood pressure, along with elevated kidney protein and liver enzymes, among other symptoms. Lastly, she reported having a considerable amount of shoulder pain and arthritis in her neck. We often see patients with chronic pain like Mary's exhibit sleep-related bruxism or clenching and grinding of teeth at night. Their pain is very stimulating, which leads to the bruxism that can be quite painful and damaging to the teeth and TM joints.

With so many health issues, it's perhaps not surprising that Mary was also depressed to the point of being under psychiatric care and taking several medications: four for anxiety, one for low thyroid, and one for chronic headaches. While Mary and her multiple issues may seem to make her an extremely challenging patient, she is an example of what I see every day in my practice.

Her sleep apnea had been diagnosed as "mild" based on a score of 8.3 on what is known as an apnea hypopnea index (AHI) or respiratory event index (REI). AHI is used when referring to an in-lab sleep test, while REI is used when referring to a home sleep test. I will go into greater detail on sleep studies later in the book. Mary's score of 8.3 meant that she was waking up and then going back to sleep more than eight times every hour during sleep. Her breathing would slow down or stop, which would wake up her brain to tell her body to start breathing again normally. Imagine what that kind of disrupted sleep does to a small child. If a child were awakened *eight times every hour* during a night of sleep, it would be pretty rough for everybody the next day. Adults are no different—they need sleep. Being disrupted constantly can wreak havoc on a person's health.

After reviewing Mary's history and discussing her victories, she underwent an evaluation to ensure that she was a good candidate for an oral appliance to treat her OSA. That evaluation included photos of her mouth and posture along with X-ray imaging of her maxilla and mandible and her airway from the tip of her nose down to her throat. The X-ray used was a cone beam computerized tomography (CBCT), which produces a three-dimensional (3-D) view of the associated structures. We use the industry's leading CBCT technology, i-CAT, which is manufactured by Imaging Sciences. It's a great tool for viewing the anatomy of the airway and the health of the temporomandibular joints (TM joint).

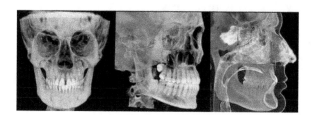

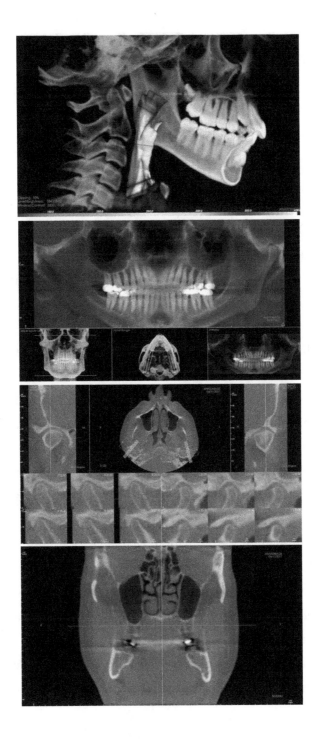

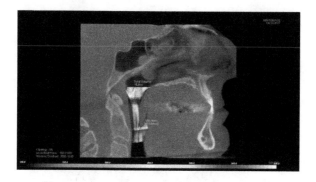

One of the challenges with Mary's treatment was that she had a small maxilla and mandible, which did not allow much room for her tongue. The tongue is a large muscle; only half of it is visible upon clinical evaluation, while the other half extends down the back of the throat. When the maxilla and mandible are narrow or pushed back, the result is limited room for the tongue. Mary's narrow features predisposed her to having an increase of a collapsing airway during the night when her body relaxed during sleep. And as her sleep test showed, her airway collapsed 8.3 times per hour, disrupting her sleep significantly. While her diagnosis was "mild" sleep apnea, it was apparent that her symptoms were far from mild.

Throughout the evaluation, Mary's victories were top of mind. By continually relating the plan for treatment back to those victories, there was a better chance that Mary would comply and follow through with every treatment aspect prescribed.

Since Mary's top victory was to do something about her frequent, heavy snoring, a symptom of OSA, the treatment plan needed to address that. As I write this book, there are more than 115 FDA-approved appliances to treat OSA, so it was important to find the one best suited to her needs.

Again, Mary had a laundry list of health problems: high blood pressure, gastroesophageal reflux (GERD), anxiety, migraines, and even depression. These were serious symptoms that were associated with her "mild" case of OSA—symptoms often mistakenly not recognized as being related. When it comes to something as serious as sleep apnea, I frequently ask patients, "What's more important than breathing, and next to breathing, what's more important than sleep?" Breathing is crucial for good sleep. Treating OSA often helps to improve, if not solve, a lot of other medical problems the patient is experiencing. I was recently at a conference with twelve hundred physicians, and a question was posed: "Why is the single most important thing to life—breathing—the thing that is evaluated least by physicians?" Well, that's not the case in my practice. Breathing is what we look at first and foremost.

Given the commitment to our new patients, the initial evaluation is very detailed, and includes a close look at medical history. Treatment only moves forward when the patient is completely on board with the plan and understands the goals along the way—the patient must truly understand their condition and own their problem. And those goals involve treating the origin of the patient's problems. Not a day goes by that when we are done with our exam a patient asks me, "Why didn't anyone else ever tell me about this?" Here, they are referring to what we discovered, learned, and diagnosed during their examination.

For Mary, the goal was to normalize her breathing, reduce her inflammation, prevent airway collapse at night, keep her breathing through her nose, and help her get quality sleep.

THERAPEUTIC VS. PALLIATIVE

Instead of just giving Mary medications to treat her symptoms and help make her comfortable, otherwise known as palliative care, her treatment plan was therapeutic in nature. It didn't involve just putting earplugs in her ears or her husband's ears to keep anyone from hearing the snore. It involved actually treating the source of her snoring—her nasal passages and unstable mandibular position.

Since Mary's nose was blocked and her mandible was collapsing back, she was getting less airflow down to her throat. Less air means a buildup of negative pressure, which causes the airway to collapse and leads to the vibrations that cause the sound of snoring. It's kind of like trying to sip a thick smoothie through a flimsy straw. Sucking on the straw with increased pressure causes it to collapse on itself greater. That's essentially what can happen when the body's muscles relax and the airway becomes flimsy and ultimately collapses.

So the solution for Mary involved stabilizing her mandible to keep it from sagging back when she relaxed during sleep. That was achieved with a 3-D-printed mandib-

ular advancement appliance, which was fitted to her upper and lower teeth. The appliance used was a Panthera D-SAD (digital sleep apnea device). It positioned her mandible in an orthopedically stable position that is proven to prevent airway collapsibility while she slept. That kept her tongue and soft palate (the tissue inside her mouth) from collapsing or sagging back during sleep, eliminating her snoring.

One of the great things about that particular appliance is its durability. Since the maxilla and mandible muscles are extremely powerful, they can create a lot of damage to the teeth when the patient clenches and grinds their teeth at night (which Mary did). Studies show that clenching and grinding during sleep is as much as five times stronger than while awake. During the day, a patient's proprioception, or awareness of their clenching forces, is controlled by their cortex (voluntary motor control). During sleep, that proprioceptive control goes to the cerebellum (the back of the brain that coordinates involuntary muscle function and activity), which allows for the production of up to five times greater force without the patient being aware of those increased forces. The Panthera D-SAD—which is made of medical-grade nylon—can withstand those forces. Yet it is extremely thin and comfortable, which made it easier for Mary to wear it nightly. It is currently the thinnest appliance in our field of practice.

Other solutions for Mary included using over-the-counter nasal spray along with Breathe Right nasal strips. Those strips adhered to her nose to open her nasal passages and

allowed her to breathe better through her nose. Dietary and lifestyle changes were also made to help five-foot-six Mary drastically reduce her weight from 190 lbs.

Again, treatment is therapeutic—most of the time. It involves digging in and addressing the source of the problem. However, sometimes treatment necessarily also involves palliative measures, or management of the symptoms instead of treating the cause. That would be the case if, for instance, someone has been in a traumatic accident and their body structures are broken, torn, or permanently damaged. Then we might only be able to manage their pain and sleep problems.

A TRUSTING RELATIONSHIP

Therapeutic treatment is ideal when rehabilitation of the problem will lead to a victory. We set expectations with our patients at their first appointment. That's when we can determine whether their treatment will be therapeutic or palliative.

We want to make sure the patient knows what to expect about their treatment and their outcomes, however, we take it slowly. With most patients, we don't attempt to explain every detail up front. In that initial visit, we only want to arm them with information. The saying "knowledge is power" is certainly true when it comes to TM joints and sleep breathing disorders (SBDs). Treatment goes beyond putting a piece of plastic in a patient's mouth and expecting it to resolve all

their problems. When we help them understand the need to be compliant (not just demand it of them), and help them see their progress along the way, they are more willing to participate in their own treatment.

But sometimes it takes a little extra explanation because many of my patients' symptoms have been around a long time and have been presented to several doctors with limited answers. For instance, when it came time to resolve Mary's headaches, I had to explain that her sleep apnea needed to be treated to resolve her head pain. Initially, she didn't understand the connection between the two, so further explanation was in order. "While sleeping," I explained, "with OSA, the body becomes deoxygenated. A classic symptom of that is morning headaches. That's because the body is more or less suffocating while sleeping, as it's being deprived of oxygen resulting in hypoxia, or the deficiency of oxygen concentration in the tissues. That results in morning headaches which is an inflammatory condition."

It comes down to a trusting relationship between the dentist and the patient. This trusting relationship helps patients be victorious, because the more they know, the more they are willing to follow the recommendations given.

MARY'S VICTORY

Just two weeks into treatment, Mary felt tremendous relief. Her snoring was gone. Her headache and shoulder pain were essentially gone, only occurring around the time of her menstrual cycle. With those levels of victories, no changes were made to her appliances, but she was still working on lifestyle changes—and she was motivated to do so because the appliance treatment was working so well.

Three months into treatment, Mary did a follow-up sleep study to validate that her OSA was treated. Sure enough, her test results came back within normal limits. Her oxygen levels were extremely good, and overall, her sleep was normalized. The sleep physician was extremely pleased with her clinical results.

She was still working on getting her weight under control, and her goal was to get off the medications she was taking for anxiety and depression.

Mary was also referred to a like-minded OB-GYN physician to help manage her menstrual cycle so that she could navigate through menopause more gracefully. Under our direction and her physicians, Mary began a low-inflammation diet, eliminating all dairy, refined or added sugar, gluten, and grains. These were recommendations specific to her conditions. She also started exercising regularly again.

As a result of Mary's treatment, she lost twenty-eight pounds in the first six months.

Ultimately, under her physician's recommendations, she was able to stop taking all her antianxiety, depression, and headache medication. These are medications she had been on for over fifteen years! Today she takes only a lower dose of thyroid medicine and some vitamins and natural supplements for overall health.

Mary is a prime example that the body wants to heal and that in the right environment, it will. Look at it this way: A cut on a person's foot will heal unless they keep walking barefoot in the mud, don't take a shower, and wear dirty socks. A cut in that environment will take a long time to heal or maybe never will.

Today, less than a year after she first came to us for treatment, Mary says she never felt better. "I'm feeling a lot better and have lots more energy," she reported. "Working with different doctors is a key to make sure you're hitting all aspects of your life, and that you're really taking care of yourself. The one important thing I learned is that I really do need to take the advice of my trusted doctors because they do know what they're talking about. And it's hard to change your life but changing my lifestyle has given me more energy and just a love of life again."

As was the case with Mary, treatment is a progression. Once we understand a patient's victory, we create a plan to address their different needs one at a time until we have them resolved. It often takes time for the body to get so ill, and it takes time for it to heal and recover. For many patients, that begins with a good night's sleep. In Mary's case, that is basically what catapulted her into the next level of overall wellness.

Today, we see Mary on an annual basis to monitor her progress and ensure that she's wearing her appliance and maintaining health. We also stay in the loop with her OB-GYN to ensure that she is achieving her victory of overall wellness.

HOLISTIC, COLLABORATIVE CARE

Why is a dentist identifying and treating conditions like these while fostering relationships for the patient with other providers such as an ear, nose, and throat physician (ENT), an OB-GYN, a naturopathic physician, and a primary care physician? Someone has to look into these problems and search for resolutions for these patients, something dentists are well positioned to do. In fact, according to a policy statement released by the American Dental Association (ADA) in 2017, "Dentists can and do play an essential role in the multidisciplinary care of patients with certain sleep related breathing disorders [SRBD] and are well positioned to identify patients at greater risk of SRBD."[2]

Care for disorders of the TM joint and for sleep apnea is holistic and collaborative; it is the bridge between medicine and dentistry, yet a little outside the typical wheelhouse of both. It took until 2007 for sleep medicine to become a recognized specialty and until 2017 for the ADA to tell dentists to look at breathing in patients. Medical physicians really don't venture into the world of chronic facial pain or maxilla and mandible pain, nor do they make oral appli-

---

2   "The Role of Dentistry in the Treatment of Sleep Related Breathing Disorders," American Dental Association, accessed April 14, 2018, https://www.ada.org/~/media/ADA/Member%20Center/Files/The-Role-of-Dentistry-in-Sleep-Related-Breathing-Disorders.pdf?la=en.

ances for OSA. The physicians we work with are screening for these disorders and identifying risk indicators for them. For several years now, I have been hosting community education events to help physicians, nurses, and dentists better understand these disorders, and it's heartwarming to see the quality of health care improving in our area.

Even though dentists can treat sleep apnea, only a board-certified sleep physician can actually diagnose it. That's just one of the medical disciplines we work with to facilitate an ideal patient outcome. Whichever discipline is involved, the message of the patient's victory is communicated to every referral provider. The patient has enough to worry about; they shouldn't have to worry about repeating their story over and over to every provider involved in their care.

Now, many ask what specialty is responsible for the TM joint. There's a long-winded history behind TMD. It was first discovered by an ENT (ear nose throat) physician, then it evolved into the realm of dentistry for treatment. So who should treat it today? The physician? The dentist? The ideal answer is both. In later chapters, I'll describe some of the origins of TMD and OSA, and you'll see how it's almost impossible for either of these providers to treat the problems alone. That's why it takes a collaborative approach from an interdisciplinary team.

Now, I routinely lecture to dentists across the country on how to better identify sleep disordered breathing for their patients. As dentists, we are in a unique position to identify some of the most common risk indicators for sleep disordered breathing. The table below illustrates and explains the relationship between these findings that every dentist should now. I firmly believe that every dentist should be identifying these clinical findings in their routine examinations.

CLINICAL FINDINGS THAT MAY INDICATE A
RISK FOR SLEEP-BREATHING DISORDERS

CLINICAL OBSERVATION	POTENTIAL RELATIONSHIP
Tongue	
Coated	Risk for gastroesophageal reflux disease or mouth breathing
Enlarged	Increased tongue activity; possible OSA
Scalloping at lateral borders (crenations)	Increased risk for sleep apnea
Obstructs view of orophrynx	Mallampati score of I and II: lower risk for OSA; Mallampati score of III and IV: increased risk for OSA
Teeth and periodontal structures	
Gingival inflammation	Mouth breather, poor oral hygiene
Gingival bleeding when probed	At risk for periodontal disease
Dry mouth (xerostomia)	Mouth breather; may be medication related
Gingival recession	May be at risk for clenching
Tooth wear	May have sleep bruxism
Abfraction (cervical abrasion/wear)	Increased parafunction/clenching
Airway	
Long sloping soft palate	At risk for OSA
Enlarged/swollen/elongated uvula	At risk for OSA/snoring

CLINICAL OBSERVATION	POTENTIAL RELATIONSHIP
Extraoral	
Chapped lips or cracking at the corners of the mouth	Inability to nose breathe
Poor lip seal; difficulty maintaining a lip seal	Chronic mouth breather
Mandibular retrognathia	Risk for OSA/snoring
Long face (doliocephalic)	Chronic mouth breathing habit
Enlarged masseter muscle	Clenching/sleep bruxism
Nose/nasal airway	
Small nostrils (nares)	Difficulty nose breathing
Alar rim collapse with forced inspiration	At risk for OSA/sleep-breathing disorder
Posture of the head/neck	
Forward head posture	Airway compromise and restriction
Loss of lordotic curve	Chronic mouth breather
Posterior rotation of the head	Tendency to mouth breathe

I've put myself in the middle between the patient and all of our referral partners to get optimum patient outcome. My job is to be the quarterback in these situations and help ensure that everybody on the team is following the game plan. And that game plan is determined by the patient's victory—the win. That's what we're all trying to accomplish.

Every patient does not have to see other providers. The cases I illustrate in this book highlight the multiple levels of symptoms we can address for our patients. Often a patient only needs to work with us. However, in some more complex cases, it really is impossible to experience a victory without that collaborative team. In upcoming chapters, I will explain the details behind these patient cases. You'll see how the practice that I've developed can help directly with many problems—

and when it can't, we can find someone who can help. That's a commitment I make to my patients: I want to give them hope to uncover the origin of their problems and get them to achieve the level of wellness they want and deserve.

CHAPTER 2
THE TRIAD OF HEALTH

Let food be thy medicine.
—Hippocrates

Before coming to see me for answers to her chronic pain, Teresa, a thirty-nine-year-old music teacher, was traveling an hour and a half for appointments to an osteopathic physician who specialized in chronic musculoskeletal pain. She had first gone to see him seven years prior and kept returning because he was able to relieve some of the debilitating neck pain that had plagued her for over thirteen years. But she still suffered from shoulder pain, headache pain, and facial pain. She fought through the pain most days, but she was finding it increasingly difficult to get through the day.

At night, Teresa had trouble falling asleep. When she was finally able to doze off, she would spend the night grinding her teeth, tossing and turning, and waking repeatedly from sleep. She never felt refreshed in the morning, and most days she had to drag herself out of bed.

Before going to the osteopathic physician, she had been to multiple providers. Solutions they had given her included a mouth guard, physical therapy, steroid injections, muscle relaxers, Lyrica (for fibromyalgia and nerve pain), prolotherapy (regenerative injections), chiropractic, and a specific blood-type diet. Surgery had also been considered, and she had even been to the Mayo Clinic for an evaluation.

Still, she found no relief. That resulted in depression, for which she had been prescribed Prozac—but that only contributed toward negative side effects.

The symptoms she reported to me when she came in for her first appointment at my practice included a constant headache and tension at the base of her skull, pain in her upper back, soreness and stiffness in both shoulders, and limited movement in her neck. Both sides of her face hurt, whether at rest or while chewing, and she reported clenching her teeth for as long as she could remember. She also had extreme pain in front of her right ear. In summing up her problems to me, she said simply, "I don't feel alive."

Teresa's victory was to eliminate her neck pain and get back to living her

—— VICTORY ——

Teresa's victory was to eliminate her neck pain and get back to living her life.

life. She did not want to be debilitated and defined by her pain, she wanted to live again.

We completed a workup on her that included photographs, 3-D imaging of the TM joints, and evaluation of her muscles and nervous system. The workup revealed some significant issues.

Part of Teresa's problem was that she had tongue-tie, where the tissue on the bottom side of her tongue was tethered to the floor of her mouth just behind her bottom front teeth. That kept her tongue from having adequate range of motion, and it pulled her head forward, which led to her neck problems.

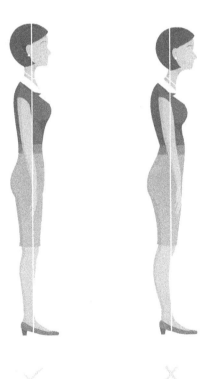

The tongue attaches to the mandible, which attaches to the first three cervical vertebrae of the neck. If the tongue and mandible are pulled forward, then we commonly see forward head posture, causing pain in the neck and back of the head.

Teresa also suffered from TMD, which was causing extreme pain around her TM joints. In fact, she had so much inflammation in her TM joints that she was unable to open her mouth all the way or chew without pain. The tests also revealed that her nasal septum was severely deviated; the bone and cartilage down the center of her nose was crooked enough to block her nasal passages, making it difficult for her to breathe. Teresa was so accustomed to the way her nose worked that she didn't even realize the difficulty she was having breathing through it. We commonly see this and it makes sense—we don't know what we don't know. I often say to patients, if we've never seen without glasses we don't know our vision is that bad until we experience it through new lenses.

As a dentist, it was tempting to look only at Teresa's physical and structural issues above the neck. However, as with all patients, there are three integrated systems that must be considered: physical/structural, chemical/nutritional, mental/spiritual. These are known as the Triad of Health.

THE TRIAD: THREE SYSTEMS OF HEALTH

Helping a patient achieve their victory is about more than simply looking inside their mouth. Since in the human body everything is interrelated, all three systems in the Triad of Health must be healthy. When one system is unhealthy, the triad is compromised. But addressing all three systems gives the patient the best chance of having the ideal environment for healing and recovery.

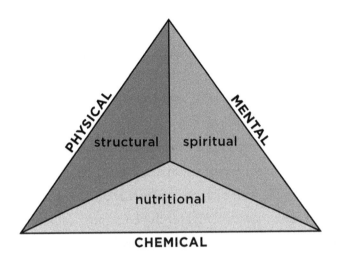

With some patients, each system of the triad is evaluated and treated concurrently, which sometimes involves partner providers. When that happens, proper education from the provider to the patient is the key to helping the patient see their problem for what it truly is.

In Teresa's case, structurally, she had the problems of tongue-tie, a deviated septum, and TMD. Those components comprised the physical/structural issues on the triad that needed to be explained to her and then treated. Her depression and suffering from pain were considered mental/spiritual issues, comprising another point on the triad. During the evaluation, Teresa actually shed a few tears when it came to discussing her mental state in dealing with her pain and depression. That's a great thing: tears shed during an exam means the patient is opening up, and that always helps us get to the heart of the problem.

The third point of the triad, the chemical/nutritional system, is something that most, if not all, patients can benefit from. The words spoken by the father of medicine, Hippocrates—"Let food be thy medicine"—were never truer than they are today, in a world where eating healthy is a challenge.

The "Triad of Health" is a phrase used in medicine to outline the three necessary systems of health. Picture an equilateral triangle, with each side of the triangle representing one of the human systems. Again, these are physical/structural, chemical/nutritional, and mental/spiritual. An imbalance in any of these areas will result in chronic inflammation, which can ultimately lead to illness or disease.

Inflammation is the precursor to all disease processes, although inflammation is not always a bad thing. The body needs inflammation to heal and recover from injuries, and that process happens day in and day out. It's when the body has too much inflammation that it starts to cause pain and wreak havoc.

The common aspect that all the systems of the triad share is that they affect the nervous system. The nervous system is king. It dictates function throughout the body, and anytime it is insulted, injured, or affected, there are negative consequences. For that reason, the nervous system guides treatment. The systems in the triad are continually evaluated throughout treatment to see whether inflammation is being created and how that is affecting the nervous system. Controlling inflammation is the primary factor in the prevention of disease, and it's vital to reversing the disease process once it is present.

Some patients have specific preexisting conditions that naturally come with chronic inflammation. Certain diseases like rheumatoid arthritis, multiple sclerosis, irritable bowel syndrome, fibromyalgia, and Lyme disease must be revealed up front or discovered during the evaluation in order to better manage their treatment.

To get a better understanding of the triad, let's look at the three systems individually.

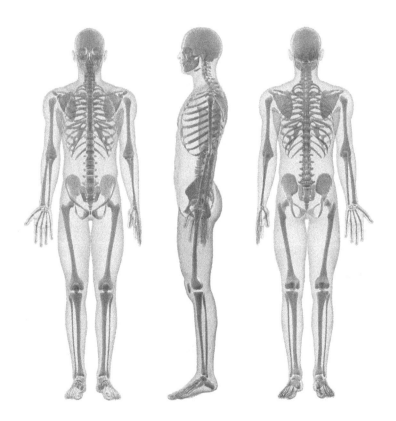

The Physical/Structural System

Humans must have a healthy physical body. For that, staying active is essential. The body must move in order to keep working well. Some experts say that at minimum, good physical health means breaking a sweat at least once a day. Some say take ten thousand steps a day. Just move—that's the key. It's important to use the body and stress the muscles enough that they're constantly building and repairing, building and repairing.

At my practice, we focus on the physical health of the TM joint and associated structures. When we talk about the physical health of most of our patients, that's the area we are evaluating.

The TM joint is interesting. It's the only joint in the body that is a bilateral diarthrodial joint, meaning that it is on both sides of the mandible and moves in several directions. Even more interesting is that the TM joints are composed of the temporal bone and the mandible, making up two joint complexes on either side of the face. Unlike other joints in the body—the knees, elbows, shoulders—the mandible as one bone connects to both joints. The right and left TM joints are connected by that one bone, the mandible, and they cannot move independently of each other.

Although the TM joints are located in the face, their health is crucial to the entire body. Any discrepancy in the joint typically causes problems not only within the joint but also in other parts of the body. The TM joints are vital for eating, breathing, and speaking—basically all things required for survival. The moment these joints become affected by inflammation, they can cause a whole host of issues. That's what was happening with Teresa and what happens with many people, as you'll see with other patient stories that I'll share.

Physical/structural health looks at the body's symmetry. Dysfunction or asymmetry in one area of the body tends to cause the body to compensate in another area. That happens because the brain cares more about survival than it does about pain. If needed, the brain will even ignore the pain and discomfort in order to keep us alive and moving. That's how someone can break a foot running out of a burning building and keep on running to get out of harm's way. It's also how people can go a long time with a chronic ailment. In spite of pain and discomfort, the brain will keep the body going in survival mode.

That survival mode, known as the sympathetic, or "fight-or-flight" state, is one of two states that the nervous system can be in. The other state is known as the parasympathetic, or "rest-and-digest" state. These terms are based on the idea that in primitive times, when humans weren't hunting or gathering food for survival, their bodies were in a parasympathetic state—resting and digesting—rejuvenating. But when in need of food or fuel, or in a fearful situation (real or perceived), their bodies reverted to survival mode—the fight-or-flight, or sympathetic state. In the sympathetic state, the heart starts racing, pupils dilate, metabolism increases, and all efforts are geared toward survival. This acute stress response leaves the patient in a state of hyperarousal.

The human body can actually go weeks without food and days without water. But it can only go minutes without air. When something obstructs the airway, the brain kicks into survival mode and the body automatically realigns its upright position to allow the lungs to breathe maximally. That's why our patient evaluation looks intently at breathing, especially the structure of the airway and the position of the body.

In addition to Teresa's tongue-tie, which caused her to position her head forward, part of the reason her neck hurt was that she couldn't breathe through her nose. Without realizing it, she was thrusting her head forward in order to breathe better, which added to the stress on her neck. That was compounded by painful TM joints and maxillary and mandibular muscles in spasm. In fact, Teresa was a little surprised that her stiff neck was not addressed first in her evaluation; no one had ever made the connection between her breathing and her neck before let alone her tongue tie which she didn't know existed. But her situation is typical of what happens with most patients who come in experiencing pain. Their brain, in survival mode, has caused some area of the body to behave in a way it is not accustomed to. As my mentor Dr. Olmos always reminds his students: "Remember, in a chronic pain situation, the site of the pain and the symptom is rarely, if ever, the origin of the problem." In Teresa's case, her obstructed airway had caused her body to shift to an unnatural position; it had compensated to keep her breathing.

That's why the evaluation focuses on the injury the patient's brain fears most. Even if the TM joint hurts, it may not be the cause of the patient's problems. That's why looking at the physical/structural health is a head-to-toe evaluation, and why treatment can involve a team of referral partners whose expertise lies in other areas of the body.

The Chemical/Nutritional System

In Hippocrates's day, medicine involved food, herbs, spices, and natural products of the earth. When people got sick, they would change their diet and alter their environment to promote healing. They knew that the body would heal if put in the right conditions.

Creating that healing environment for patients means having the inflammation needed to heal, but not so much inflammation that it's causing destruction. For instance, when a patient is trying to heal, they need a healthy environment. A person who has a terrible diet and who smokes and drinks alcohol to excess certainly won't heal as quickly as someone who has a healthy diet and avoids smoking and alcohol. It's like the foot analogy I mentioned in the last chapter: If a person gets a cut on their foot and then walks barefoot through mud and doesn't clean the cut afterward, it's less likely to heal than if they wash it and keep it clean and isolated.

Food can produce inflammation that can wreak havoc in the body. Just as taking a dose of Advil can decrease inflammation, a teaspoon of sugar can increase inflammation. That teaspoon of sugar may not be labeled "inflammatory," but like much of the food available today, it can make a significant difference in how a person feels.

In this age of processed foods and additives and other inflammatory ingredients (such as sugar), it is a challenge to fuel the body with high-quality natural food—a good mix of fruits, vegetables, and proteins. Put it this way: If you bought a high-performance vehicle—a Mercedes, for instance—would you fill it with premium or low-graded fuel? You'd want to use premium gas on such a sophisticated machine. Well, your body is much more sophisticated, and it needs the best fuel to keep running efficiently. If you google the work of Dr. Robert Lustig, a pediatric endocrinologist, you will learn an enormous amount about how what we eat affects our livelihood and well-being. That topic is a book in and of itself.

Another aspect of the chemical/nutritional system is getting adequate sleep. Sleep is essential for the brain to rest, heal, and recover from the day's activities. An amazing number of chemical processes happen in the body and bloodstream during sleep, basically resetting the body. It's important to create an environment that allows for seven to nine hours of sleep each night so that the body and brain can heal and be ready for the next day. Children require much more sleep than this as they are growing and developing.

Good sleep relies, in part, on the nutrition a person gets throughout the day. Guiding a patient's nutrition during treatment can involve working with a specialist, such as a nurse practitioner, nutritionist, dietitian, or wellness coach to evaluate diet deficiencies and what's needed to correct those. We offer these services as part of treatment and have relationships with many providers in the community to ensure that we can help get our patients what they need.

AGE	RECOMMENDED	NOT RECOMMENDED
Newborns *0-3 months*	14-17 hours	Less than 11 hours More than 19 hours
Infants *4-11 months*	12-15 hours	Less than 10 hours More than 18 hours
Toddlers *1-2 years*	11-14 hours	Less than 9 hours More than 16 hours
Preschoolers *3-5 years*	10-13 hours	Less than 8 hours More than 14 hours
School-Aged Children *6-13 years*	9-11 hours	Less than 7 hours More than 12 hours
Teenagers *14-17 years*	8-10 hours	Less than 7 hours More than 11 hours
Young Adults *18-25 years*	7-9 hours	Less than 6 hours More than 11 hours

The Mental/Spiritual System

The mental/spiritual system in the triad is about the patient's overall mental stability and happiness in life. Often, patients are simply worn down by the chronic physical/structural problems, sleep problems, and overall health issues they are experiencing. It's common to see patients who are dealing with anxiety, frustration, and depression.

Good healing relies in part on a patient being in good spirits and mentally fit. That starts by letting the patient know that it's understandable that they're in poor spirits. In fact, when I see a patient dealing with so much chronic pain, I give them permission to have those feelings—I'd probably be in poor spirits, too, if I were dealing with the same issues for so long.

Part of every provider's role is to instill hope. Dr. Mark Cantieri, a doctor I look up to, a friend and world-renowned osteopathic physician, once said to me, "Hope is the one thing that every provider can give his or her patient—don't ever take that away from a patient." It takes effort to heal from temporomandibular joint disorders (TMD) and sleep breathing disorders (SBD). Once a patient understands the reasons for their problems and realizes that there are potential solutions, some of them immediately begin to feel better—even before treatment begins. That's because hope is a powerful virtue; on its own, it can actually start the therapeutic process.

When needed, a patient may be referred to a psychologist or psychiatrist for a bit of added help and to ensure that the mental/spiritual system is being effectively addressed. We refer patients to these providers when the initial evaluation reveals emotional, physical, verbal, and/or sexual abuse, as these are not our areas of expertise but can play a huge part in a patient's overall well-being.

Obviously, the mental/spiritual system can be especially sensitive for patients, so being respectful of their situation is key. Still, this system is a necessary part of the triad, and it is crucial that it be addressed to ensure victory. Fixing the physical/structural system alone won't ensure victory, nor will focusing solely on the chemical/nutritional system. For healing—and a victory—to occur, the patient must have a sound body, mind, and spirit.

TERESA'S VICTORY

As stated, all three systems in the triad must be evaluated to determine the primary problem before a treatment plan is created. Although Teresa had consulted with very good practitioners, her problems had been treated in the wrong order. Since her primary physical problem turned out to be her breathing—her nose was obstructed and her tongue was tied down—those physical and structural components had to be addressed before she could see progress toward her victory. After all, nothing trumps breathing!

Once her nasal obstruction was conservatively addressed by an ENT, and her tongue-tie was released with a mild laser procedure, Teresa's breathing was restored and she experienced a cascade of improvement. After that, her jaw pain and facial pain were corrected using intraoral orthotics, appliances that specifically position the maxilla and mandible in a neurologically orthopedically stable position to allow for healing. These are very different from splints, which are static appliances that simply cover the teeth in a non-positioned manner.

On her mandibular teeth, Teresa wore a daytime appliance for twelve weeks to heal her joints. During that same time frame, she wore a different orthotic at nighttime to help facilitate proper breathing through her nose and to keep her airway from collapsing while she slept. Her TM joints were treated like they had a stress fracture or a bad sprain. They were held in an orthopedically stable position to allow them to heal and inflammation to subside.

The orthotic also helped her head become upright on her spine, relieving her neck pain. Research conducted in 2005 by Dr. Olmos explains that treatment of TM joint dysfunction will upright the head posture by 4.43 inches on average for patients like Teresa, while improving the orthopedic stability of the TM joint.[3] It is fortunate that Teresa never pursued neck surgery, which was recommended by a previous provider, because that wouldn't have resolved the issue since her neck wasn't the primary problem. We proved this by resolving her neck pain without touching her neck—it

---

3   Olmos, Steven, et al., "The Effect of Condyle Fossa Relationships on Head Posture," *The Journal of Craniomandibular Practice* 23, no. 1 (January 2005): 48–52.

sounds crazy at first, but makes total sense when you understand the entire picture.

Dietary changes were also part of Teresa's treatment plan to ensure that inflammation was reduced from the start. With some patients, inflammation must be reduced before they can begin to see other providers for treatment. Reducing inflammation can allow the body's immune system to regain functionality, which can help the patient's own body heal some of the issues they are experiencing. Eliminating inflammatory foods from the diet is one of the quickest ways to begin that process.

In addition to the physical/structural and chemical/nutritional issues that Teresa was dealing with, her treatment included visiting with a psychologist to deal with the mental aspects of what she had been going through for thirteen years. For instance, she had shared with us that, with previous treatments, she would wake up in the morning some days and tell her husband, "This is the day they're going to tell me they can't help me anymore, so just be prepared when I get home." Her fear and dread weren't because her pain was particularly worse that day. It was because she felt that hope would be taken away and she might have to live with her pain. That's the power of hope and it's role in healing. This is what Dr. Cantieri was educating me about early on.

Teresa's treatment required help from multiple providers. At one point, there was a brief hurdle that had her concerned that we were going to "break up" with her. But we found an additional provider to help her overcome that hurdle.

After living with chronic and increasing pain for thirteen years without any solution, it took a village to help Teresa be completely pain-free. The bulk of her issues were resolved in only four months; it was worth every minute for Teresa. "I am pain free for the first time in nearly thirteen years and loving life, just enjoying being able to do whatever I want to do," she said.

Her advice to other people in pain and without answers? "You need to just do it," she said. "You have absolutely nothing to lose in coming in and getting a consult and seeing what can be done for you, because it can be life changing."

Teresa's video testimonial and hundreds of others are on our website at www.tmjsleep-indiana.com/testimonials.

As I've mentioned, getting to the root of the problem means looking in depth at the patient's medical history. Often, helping patients overcome chronic pain is like peeling away the layers of an onion, with each layer helping to manage all the components of care on their road to victory. Like you saw with Teresa, there were many steps leading her back to a path of increased overall wellness—and the longer you put it off or continue chronically treating your chronic pain, the longer it takes for you to get to the source of your problems and start healing ... for good.

In the next chapter, I'll talk about what it means to treat patients' issues layer after layer.

CHAPTER 3
THE IMPORTANCE OF FINDING THE SOURCE— ESPECIALLY FOR ATHLETES

There is nothing sudden about a heart attack; it takes years of preparation.

Thirty-nine-year-old Justin was a busy business executive from Milwaukee, Wisconsin, who was in town for work when a colleague suggested he come see me. He was an ultra-distance marathon runner who was training for a fifty-mile run through the woods. However, his times had been getting slower, because he'd been having chronic knee and hip pain for about six months, hindering his training.

He wasn't taking any medications but was under the care of a chiropractor and receiving treatments weekly to attempt to stay ahead of his knee and hip pain. He'd been to an orthopedic surgeon and various other doctors, who had tried foot orthotics, stretching exercises, and different modalities, but nothing had really been able to kick the knee pain. Justin wasn't sure what was causing it, and his doctors were also baffled. Pretty much everyone chalked his problems up to his running, believing he was probably just pushing himself too hard. But Justin was committed to being in an ultramarathon, so he was working through the pain.

Admittedly, Justin was reluctant to see a dentist about knee and hip pain, but his colleague explained that we see chronic pain patients and our goal is to get to the source of the problem, figure out what's wrong and who can help, and then provide a treatment plan to help patients get better.

Justin's victory was to eliminate his hip and knee pain and feel better while running. Initially, we explained that his knee and hip pain could potentially be related to his chronic breathing issues revealed in his medical history, or to the clicking and popping within his TM joints.

—— VICTORY ——

Justin's victory was to eliminate his hip and knee pain and feel better while running.

Justin agreed to undergo a comprehensive exam. The exam would allow us to determine the three things that all patients want to know:

1. What's wrong?

2. What can we do to help?

3. How long will treatment take?

The exam revealed substantial findings. The evaluation of his posture showed that he had extreme forward head position and his feet were divergent, basically pointing outward, like a duck. When the head is postured forward, the feet must be divergent in order to hold the body upright. Poor balance will result in forward head posture, leading to structural decompensation. In addition, every inch that the head is forward puts an extra ten pounds of weight on the spine—that's the basic physics of these situations.

Forward head posture like Justin had is commonly associated with chronic nasal obstruction and craniofacial pain. An examination of his head and neck muscles revealed that they were extremely tender, specifically around the TM joints. He wasn't even aware of how painful they were but applying only three to five pounds of pressure to specific areas revealed significant discomfort.

In Justin's case, it seemed likely that his chronic forward head posture was the culprit for his knee and hip pain—aka postural decompensation. Again, since the body has the innate ability to compensate for other structural injuries, it can produce symptoms that seem unrelated but are actually connected in some way. Postural decompensation is the improper distribution of our body weight resulting from maladaptation of the normal mechanisms for homeostasis. Thus, one ailment produces improper posture and that decompensation produces additional problems like a domino effect. The extra weight of that forward head position required Justin's body to deal with unbalanced forces as he was running, and it wasn't until he began stressing his body for the ultramarathon that the imbalance began to cause noticeable pain.

Justin's case demonstrates why posture photos are an important part of the intake process. Those photos help identify how a patient's skeleton is bearing the weight of their bones while in a standing position. Imaging of the TM joints is also crucial, helping to reveal whether there is osteoarthritis in the joint or potential dysfunction of the airway passages. When we image TM joints, we acquire data of the facial structures between the TM joints, so we see the anatomy of the face, nasal passages, and sinus cavities. Justin's imaging illustrated a chronic sinus infection, a deviated nasal septum, and a bone spur of his left nasal passage. These were causing him to have a chronic nasal obstruction, which was causing his forward head posture.

By digging a little deeper, we found that Justin also had gastroesophageal reflux (GERD), or heartburn, which he had tried to remedy with dietary changes. GERD can also be a symptom of mouth breathing or an obstruction of the airway. When a person chronically breathes through their mouth, it can dry out the airway, leading to irritation. Mouth breathing can also lower the body's pH and cause negative pressure that pulls up the acid contents of the stomach, causing GERD. Now, there are numerous causes for GERD. In my evaluation, I simply

want to rule out or confirm that the cause is under my area of expertise. After explaining that to Justin, he disclosed that he was a chronic mouth breather, something he always thought was normal since he had never really breathed through his nose. Patients commonly adapt to what seems "normal" when they have never experienced what actually is normal and healthy. "Since you've never breathed through anybody else's nose, you can't be expected to know what is normal and healthy. You only know what you've experienced yourself," I explained to him. After all, we only know what we know, and we don't know what we don't know.

Justin's situation is similar to what often happens in life. An analogy I like to use is that of changing the oil in the car. That should be done every five to ten thousand miles. If the oil change is delayed to, say, twenty thousand miles, the car may continue to run "fine" without any noticeable problems—until it breaks down and leaves you stranded on the side of the road. Once the car is in the hands of the mechanic, he or she will open the hood, look inside, and identify the problem. On the outside, the car seems fine, but under the hood there's a problem—maybe even multiple problems, since the oil change was delayed for so long. Yes, it was running "fine" on Tuesday, but Wednesday, when it ended up in front of trained eyes, the longstanding problems could be identified rather quickly.

Justin had several problems "under the hood," so to speak, but until he had appreciable symptoms, he just kept on going. That's why the phrase "There's nothing sudden about a heart attack" often rings so true. Until a person is privy to what's brewing under the surface—until a physician warns them that they have high blood pressure that needs to be addressed—they'll keep on going with the busyness of their life, never realizing that they have cardiovascular disease.

Health problems are often asymptomatic (lacking symptoms) until pain or a disruption in life occurs. Take cavities, for instance. Until a cavity becomes symptomatic or painful, it usually goes undetected by the patient. That's why dentists periodically take X-rays. They want to identify cavities in order to catch them early, before they start to cause pain. Early identification can alleviate the need for a root canal or having a tooth pulled. This same early identification rings true for temporomandibular joint disorders (TMD) and sleep breathing disorders (SBD).

LOOKING UNDER THE HOOD

As a trained professional, the TM joint specialist's job is to look under the hood, see what's brewing, and try to identify the origin of the problem. Identifying the origin of the problem is the best way to get sustained relief. Dr. Olmos says that an accurate diagnosis is 95 percent of effective treatment. That's the only way to know exactly what to treat and the only way to achieve a patient's victory. That's why the intake process with patients is extremely detailed and involves the medical history and the journey the patient has been on. Every day, patients tell me they truly appreciate our thoroughness and did not expect us to go into such great detail.

Another reason for taking a deep dive into a patient's medical history is to build trust and rapport. I need to hear the patient's story. That helps patients relax and feel comfortable enough to reveal background information that they may have thought irrelevant to their problem. A relationship built on trust helps surface sensitive issues such as eating disorders, depression, suicide attempts, and other medical concerns that have been building for a long time. Getting permission from the patient to understand and learn about those allows for a more accurate diagnosis and a better treatment plan, allowing providers to be a better resource for patients. I, for one, feel honored when a patient shares a painful experience with me. It motivates me to help care for them better and to work ceaselessly to ensure they get accurate treatment, whether with my office or with another provider.

Getting to the source of the problem is why the first evaluation takes an hour or more, and why the clinical exam is so comprehensive. That comprehensive exam helps identify all the underlying issues that may be related to the patient's symptoms.

Again, with chronic conditions, the site or location of the pain is often not the origin of the problem. Dr. John Beck, an orthopedic surgeon, wrote: "Chronic pain symptoms are often trade-offs the brain is willing to make to protect a higher priority life process. Simply stated, pain is not a survival priority in nature."[4]

Chronic pain is usually a functional condition. In Dr. Beck's opinion, medicine has come to rely too much on radiological and electrodiagnostic technology and not enough on testing based on how the body functions. Novice physicians just entering practice quickly learn that back pain encompasses far more problems than answers using the standard methods of diagnosis. That's why evaluation of chronic conditions must look at the patient's functionality. It needs to consider how the person walks (their gait), their posture when standing, and how the nervous system reacts to different kinds of stimulus.

To evaluate the nervous system, Dr. Beck devised a series of tests of neurological reflexes known as autonomic motor nerve reflex testing (AMNRT). These are tests of the autonomic nervous system, which controls the internal organs such as the heart, lungs, stomach, and kidneys. The autonomic nervous system is composed of the sympathetic (fight-or-flight) and parasympathetic (rest-and-digest) systems, which I discussed in Chapter 2.[5] The reflexes are used to identify the primary structural instability, which

4   Beck, John L., "Practical Application of Neuropostural Evaluations, The P.A.N.E. Process: Basic Principles and the First Three Tests," *Practical Pain Management* 8, issue 7 (September 2008): 47–53.

5   Low, Phillip, "Overview of the Autonomic Nervous System," Merck Manual, accessed April 14, 2018, https://www.merckmanuals.com/home/brain,-spinal-cord,-and-nerve-disorders/autonomic-nervous-system-disorders/overview-of-the-autonomic-nervous-system.

helps determine which health professional needs to assist the patient.

In Justin's case, motor nerve reflex testing illustrated that his TM joints were the primary cause of his structural instability, which meant that appliance therapy was the best place to start in solving his problems. That's based on Dr. Olmos' findings that I mentioned in the previous chapter, about treatment for TMD pain and TM joint pain using intraoral orthotic therapy to upright the head posture an average 4.43 inches.[6] In other words, by correcting the position of the TM joints through orthotic therapy, the head is able to move back over the spine, reducing pain and inflammation in other areas of the body while improving breathing.

WHERE THE PROBLEM LIES

As I've mentioned, patients often come to us for what they believe is a specific problem, only to find that their pain is coming from somewhere else in their body. For instance, a patient's back or knee pain may actually be caused by problems in the TM joints. Conversely, chronic facial pain may actually be caused by an injury to the foot, back, or neck. The pain in their face is only a symptom; the injury to their back is the real source of the problem.

The intake and evaluation processes are about acknowledging the patient's pain, identifying all their issues, and then

---

6   Olmos, Steven, et al., "The Effect of Condyle Fossa Relationships on Head Posture," *The Journal of Craniomandibular Practice* 23, no. 1 (January 2005): 48–52.

giving them hope that there's a solution for their problems. That can be a struggle for the patient to comprehend. For instance, if they come in for jaw pain, and the evaluation instead seems to center on their nasal passages, they sometimes grow frustrated because they feel their concerns are being overlooked. But consider it from this angle: If water is dripping from the kitchen ceiling, that's what the homeowner will want repaired. But if a handyman finds that the leak is coming from a hole in the roof, then patching the kitchen ceiling isn't fixing the problem unless the hole in the roof is also fixed. That means calling in a roofer to do their share of the repairs first, and then patching the kitchen ceiling.

Like the roof, it often takes a team to deliver a sustained victory for patients. That's what it took in Justin's case. Since he was diagnosed as having nasal congestion, during treatment he was referred to an ENT physician who started him on over-the-counter sinus rinses and nasal sprays.

JUSTIN'S VICTORY

Justin's primary problem was determined to be capsulitis of the TM joints (inflammation of the joint capsule), which led to his chronic forward head posture. His nasal obstruction was at the heart of the issue as well. To rehabilitate and reduce the inflammation and clicking noise in his TM joints and help him learn to breathe through his nose instead of his mouth, he underwent decompression orthotic therapy, which required him to wear daytime and nighttime orthotics for twelve weeks. Those appliances stabilized his maxilla and mandible by placing them in a neurologically orthopedic position and helped upright his head on his spine to stabilize his posture. He also wore the daytime orthotic while running and while working out, which were the times he was putting the most force on his TM joints.

Just three weeks after receiving his orthotics, Justin reported that his sleep had dramatically improved. As with his mouth breathing, Justin thought that his sleep was fine; he didn't even realize it was subpar. Now that he breathes better while sleeping, he is able to sleep more soundly and feels far more rested when he wakes up. He is also able to breathe better while running, because he regularly uses a sinus rinse and wears a Breathe Right strip when he runs.

At his three-week evaluation, his head posture had also uprighted, alleviating his knee pain and jaw clicking, and nearly alleviating his hip pain. After twelve weeks, he had no hip pain and he was running better than ever—beating all of his previous times. He no longer needed physical therapy, massage therapy, or chiropractic care.

The Saturday before that twelve-week visit, he ran twenty miles, a distance that would normally have made him rest for the remainder of the day. Instead, he was able to go home after his run, play with his kids, and even mow the lawn. The next day he was a little sore, but he was able to function fully without taking the day off. "I definitely feel like the treatment has helped improve my running (and) my breathing," he said.

Treating the TM joint dysfunction and uprighting the head posture made a significant difference for Justin.[7] Had his TM joints and chronic sinus disease not been accurately identified as the cause of his forward head posture, and his forward head posture as the cause of his hip and knee pain, then dental treatments would not have provided him answers. Instead, just a couple of weeks into treatment it was apparent that the appliance therapy was the best solution—and the results were amazing.

It's surprising how often we see situations like Justin's in our office. As TM joint and sleep specialists, patients often report having chronic facial pain, headaches, dizziness, blurred vision, and other symptoms that they don't think are related to the TM joints. But the problems of the TM joints manifest in numerous craniofacial symptoms above and below the neck. Getting to the origin of a problem is the approach we take with every single patient.

In the next chapter, I'll discuss how millions of people in the United States suffer from these TM joint problems, and many of them go undiagnosed.

---

7   Olmos, Steven, et al., "The Effect of Condyle Fossa Relationships on Head Posture," *The Journal of Craniomandibular Practice* 23, no. 1 (January 2005): 48–52.

CHAPTER 4
TMJ—THE GREAT IMPOSTER

Over ten million people in the United States suffer from TM joint problems.
—The National Institutes of Health

Although Rick was a forty-year-old medical professional who oversaw sports performance, player development, and overall wellness for athletes at a multimillion-dollar operation, he struggled to figure out why he had poor sleep quality and quantity. At night, he had trouble falling asleep, and he would often spend the night tossing and turning. After such a restless night, he rarely woke feeling refreshed. Worse, he often woke with neck pain and had headaches that sometimes lasted for days. He also had ringing in his ears and a chronic sore throat accompanied by the constant feeling that he had a foreign object in his throat.

His medical history indicated that he had atrial fibrillation (AFib), an irregular and often rapid heartbeat that can increase the risk of stroke, heart failure, and other heart-related complications. AFib is when the upper two chambers of the heart beat out of sync, resulting in heart palpitations, shortness of breath, and weakness. Obstructive sleep apnea (OSA) is known to be associated with AFib, something we keep in mind as we evaluate patients with symptoms like Rick's. His AFib stemmed from a diagnosis of supraventricular tachycardia (SVT), an abnormally fast heart rhythm for which he was taking the medication Flecainide. Rick also suffered from chronic allergies for which he took allergy medications and used two different nasal sprays.

Rick's health problems had begun to disrupt his daily routine for himself and his family. His victory was to improve his sleep quality and quantity to get back some sense of normalcy in his life.

—— VICTORY ——

Rick's victory was to improve his sleep quality and quantity to get back some sense of normalcy in his life.

In examining Rick, I felt right away that even though he was reporting sleep to be his problem, many of his symptoms were related to a disorder of the TM joints. Chronic, recurrent headaches and facial pain are quite common and affect up to 20 percent of the population, according to the National Institutes of Health.[8] But people with TMD also commonly report ear symptoms such as pain, ringing, or buzzing along with clicking and popping of the TM joints. Historically, these symptoms appear to be unrelated, which is why they are often treated by multiple doctors, all of whom fail to address the origin of the problem. Symptoms like Rick was experiencing are commonly misdiagnosed as migraine or tension-type headaches, stress, or inflammation or pain associated with nerves (neuritis or neuralgia). Unfortunately, when treatment for these various conditions fails, patients are often labeled as hypochondriacs and told "It's all in your head." Even worse, these patients aren't taken seriously or are just abandoned.

TMD—A COMPLEX DIAGNOSIS

TM joint symptoms can be vast and complex. In fact, they are so challenging to understand that patients commonly go from doctor to doctor, only to end up frustrated because they haven't received any real help. If they do receive some relief, their symptoms usually return because the underlying cause is not treated.

When a patient presents with common signs and symptoms of TMD, we start looking at whether they are

---

8   "Prevalence of TMJD and its Signs and Symptoms," Research, National Institute of Dental and Craniofacial Research, last modified February 2018, https://www.nidcr.nih.gov/research/data-statistics/facial-pain/prevalence

independent symptoms from various, unrelated disorders or a compilation of symptoms from one disorder.

Let me take a moment to clarify some misconceptions about craniofacial pain, TMJ, and TMD. Craniofacial pain is exceptional, debilitating pain and discomfort in the head and face that can significantly affect a person's quality of life. This kind of pain is more than the occasional headache requiring Advil or Tylenol to provide relief.

DO YOU SUFFER FROM ANY OF THE FOLLOWING?

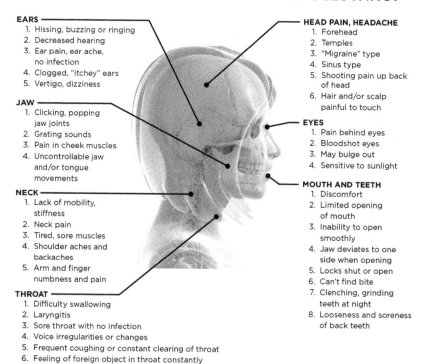

EARS
1. Hissing, buzzing or ringing
2. Decreased hearing
3. Ear pain, ear ache, no infection
4. Clogged, "itchy" ears
5. Vertigo, dizziness

JAW
1. Clicking, popping jaw joints
2. Grating sounds
3. Pain in cheek muscles
4. Uncontrollable jaw and/or tongue movements

NECK
1. Lack of mobility, stiffness
2. Neck pain
3. Tired, sore muscles
4. Shoulder aches and backaches
5. Arm and finger numbness and pain

THROAT
1. Difficulty swallowing
2. Laryngitis
3. Sore throat with no infection
4. Voice irregularities or changes
5. Frequent coughing or constant clearing of throat
6. Feeling of foreign object in throat constantly

HEAD PAIN, HEADACHE
1. Forehead
2. Temples
3. "Migraine" type
4. Sinus type
5. Shooting pain up back of head
6. Hair and/or scalp painful to touch

EYES
1. Pain behind eyes
2. Bloodshot eyes
3. May bulge out
4. Sensitive to sunlight

MOUTH AND TEETH
1. Discomfort
2. Limited opening of mouth
3. Inability to open smoothly
4. Jaw deviates to one side when opening
5. Locks shut or open
6. Can't find bite
7. Clenching, grinding teeth at night
8. Looseness and soreness of back teeth

As I mentioned at the beginning of the book, the TMJ refers to the temporomandibular joints, which are located on each side of the face. Everyone has TMJ—in fact, we all have two TMJs, a left one and a right one. When patients say, "I have TMJ," what they truly mean is that they have a *disorder* or *dysfunction* of the TMJ. To avoid confusion, I often use the term "TM joint" when I'm talking about the anatomical structure of the temporomandibular joint versus TMD, the disorder that affects the joint.

The TM joint is a truly unique joint in that it is actually two joint spaces encompassing one bone. The two joint spaces are on each side of the face, and the bone connecting the two is the mandible. The joint spaces consist of the condyle of the mandible, which sits within the glenoid fossa of the temporal bone, creating what is known as the TM joint complex.

In regard to the TM joints, one joint cannot move without influencing the other. The joint is intended to move within and out of the glenoid fossa to allow the person to speak and eat. The glenoid fossa is the space in the temporal bone of the skull where the mandible rests. The top portion of the mandible is called the condyle. The joint should allow the mouth to open vertically forty-two to fifty-two millimeters, and the mandible should be able to move laterally, side to side, about twelve to fourteen millimeters. The mandible should also be able to move forward about eight millimeters.

Although the two TM joints move as one, they can differ in shape, size, and function. Furthermore, since they're connected, there can be a problem on one side that may not have the same symptoms in the other side. In fact, pain can start on one side of the head and migrate to the other side.

Lastly, inside the TM joint is a cartilaginous structure called the articular disc, located between the condyle and the glenoid fossa. The articular disc is attached to muscle at the front end, which allows it to move forward with the condyle as it moves within and out of the glenoid fossa. On the back end, it is attached by connective tissue that helps keep the articular disc stabilized and secure.

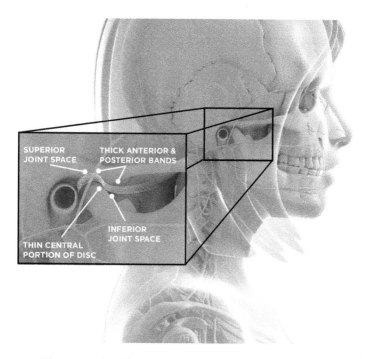

The articular disc is a shock absorber between the two bones. Since the ligaments that hold it in place are elastic, they can be stretched, causing the articular disc to be mal-positioned or moved out of place, causing many problems. Improper positioning of the articular disc can result in pain, limited opening and movement, clicking, popping, and crepitus, which is a gravel-type sound indicating bone-on-bone contact during function.

Remember: The TM joint is not like any other. It is not a ball-and socket joint like other joints in the body, which move in a hinge-like fashion, many with a ball pivoting inside a socket. The jaw joint is multidimensional. The condyle moves in and out of the glenoid fossa (the socket of the temporal bone, or skull). This is why the TM joint is referred to as a bilateral diarthroidal joint. It is meant to move in and out of the socket and laterally while being connected to another joint space—two joints, one common bone.

TMD is a group of maladies that affect the TM joints, the muscles of the jaw, neck, and face, and associated neurologic and vascular structures. Commonly these disorders are caused by injuries resulting from macro or micro trauma or inherited genetic factors. Macro trauma would be an accident with a considerable force, such as a blow to the face, a car accident, whiplash, or a fall. Micro trauma includes repetitive and recurrent exacerbation of muscle spasms resulting in increased forces on the TM joints and the associated structures. Micro traumas comprise the majority of what we see and treat in clinical practice.

Problems within and around the joint complex produce an array of symptoms that on the surface appear to be unrelated to the TM joints. These symptoms often include:

- ☐ Headache pain
- ☐ Ear pain
- ☐ Jaw pain
- ☐ Chewing pain
- ☐ Face pain
- ☐ Eye pain
- ☐ Throat pain
- ☐ Neck pain
- ☐ Shoulder pain
- ☐ Back pain
- ☐ Limited ability to open mouth
- ☐ Difficulty closing mouth
- ☐ Jaw joint locking
- ☐ Jaw joint noises
- ☐ Stuffiness
- ☐ Sinus congestion
- ☐ Dizziness
- ☐ Ringing in the ears
- ☐ Muscle spasms
- ☐ Vision problems
- ☐ Numbness

Patients do not always present with all the symptoms of TMD, but oftentimes more symptoms exist than the patient is even aware of, since the brain prioritizes pain in the order it is affecting survival. I'm often impressed with the tolerance to pain and discomfort many of my patients are experiencing.

METHODS FOR DIAGNOSING TMD

As stated earlier, 95 percent of effective treatment is accurate diagnosis, and accurate diagnosis only comes from a proper review of medical history and review of bodily systems followed by a comprehensive evaluation. Dr. Olmos devised an amazing system for evaluating the TM joints and associated structures. In my opinion, his system is second to none; it is the most thorough examination process available for evaluating these structures.

Our examination process is our way of looking for real proof that we can help. Before starting treatment, we want proof that we aren't just taking a shot in the dark, but that we have evidence that the presenting symptoms are related to the conditions that we, in fact, can treat and alleviate. I take my job very seriously, and when I tell a patient I can help them, I want to be certain that I can help them. Too many patients with chronic pain have been told by too many providers that they can be helped—and yet they arrive at our office with pain.

The best part about Dr. Olmos's system is that it is ever evolving and updated as we progress as a profession. I have the honor of collaborating with him on research projects and continuing educations for other medical providers. In additional to lecturing, part of the reason I travel so much now is to attend courses on the updates in the medical environment.

Since the TMJ, a.k.a. the "great imposter," is so complex and can lead to mysterious symptoms, it can be a tricky structure to evaluate and treat. Many of the symptoms that patients are suffering from can actually be problems of the TM joint in disguise. It is best to start from a position of higher prognosis certainty so that we don't rush the evaluation and examination process and make assumptions.

The brain devotes a great deal of neurologic support to the mouth, nose, throat, and jaw structures, because these are all needed for survival—breathing, drinking, and eating. The amount of brain devoted to certain body parts for survival can be seen in our friend here, the "cortical homunculus," which illustrates graphically the amount of brain devoted to specific body parts. It is not surprising that those involved with breathing, eating, and drinking are the largest, since they are what allow us to continue to exist. If something is off in those areas, a lot of alarms can signal there's a problem.

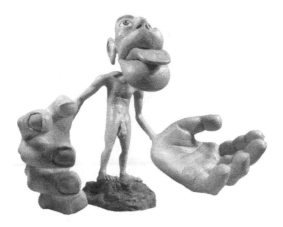

An evaluation of the TM joint complex looks first at orthopedic ranges of motion of the jaw and neck to ensure that function is within normal limits. It's similar to seeing an orthopedic surgeon about a knee or shoulder problem—the first thing they're going to evaluate is range of motion to ensure that the joints can move as intended. Joints remain healthy by adequate range of the motion, which allows fluid to constantly move throughout the joint space cavity, nourishing it.

Next, we evaluate and document all anatomic structures, noting any variations from the norm. A physical exam includes the jaws, teeth, tongue, muscles surrounding the structures, and the nasal and sinus passages. After all, the bottom half or floor of the nose is the top half of the maxilla. We also evaluate the ears, since the ear canal rests right up against the TM joint complex.

Since nine of the twelve cranial nerves pass through the TM joint and control over 125 different muscles, it is also important to evaluate these nerves. A discrepancy of one of these nerves could be a sign of problems inside the head or of a tumor compressing these nerves as they exit the cranium. Unfortunately, we have found that to be the case in rare circumstances, so intracranial pathology must be ruled out.

We then evaluate any friction within the TM joints with what is known as joint vibration analysis (JVA). JVA is an invaluable tool for evaluating TM joint function and for diagnosing pathology of the TM joints. Traditionally, a stethoscope or Doppler was used to hear joint sounds, but those rely on the hearing ability of the examiner, which can result in shortcomings. JVA passively listens to and records the vibrations of the TM joints while in motion. We want smooth gliding surfaces within the joint space, and the JVA allows us to document the friction upon movement. Those objective recordings are then used to help evaluate dysfunction of the TM joints.

Clinical studies have found that the JVA is superior to the stethoscope or Doppler for evaluation of joint noises. Furthermore, all TM joint noises (popping/clicking/crepitus) are pathologic, indicating disease or dysfunction, but even joints that are quiet are not necessarily normal and healthy. Thus, JVA is merely a piece of the comprehensive clinical exam that leads to the most accurate diagnosis and effective treatment.

Evaluation of posture and the condition of the teeth are also extremely important for effective diagnosis. Oftentimes, patient posture is affected by longstanding injuries or difficulty with proper breathing. Over time, these can lead to the postural decompensation I defined earlier. The first rule of CPR (cardiopulmonary resuscitation) is to tilt the head and lift the chin (head tilt chin lift)—this elongates the neck to improve the airway. When the posture of the head is forward, it can produce problems all the way down the spine into the lower back. The old song about the head bone being connected to the tail bone is accurate—a change in the upper portion of the spine inevitably causes changes at the base of it. By comparing before-and-after photographs, we can see just how much improvement a patient is making as they progress through treatment.

After all the aforementioned information is gathered, if clinically indicated, we image the TM joints and associated structures using CBCT, a vital tool for evaluating the hard tissue structures and airway. In the past, plain film or two-dimensional radiography was the best tool available, but it had numerous shortcomings because it could not image the structures in 3-D. These images are referred to as Panoramic X-rays, PANO's, or Panorex. The CBCT's 3-D images allow us to see variations in the anatomy and provide way more information needed for a proper diagnosis and treatment plan.

Low-dose imaging using CBCT has been a real game changer in the TMD and sleep profession. The "dose" in CBCT refers to the radiological units that are absorbed by the body during the imaging process. These dose units are known as microsieverts (μSv). It is common practice to minimize exposure to radiation. That means only taking images that are absolutely necessary in formulating a diagnosis and ensuring that the exposure is not going to cause harm. CT (computerized tomography) images at the hospital emit up to 10,000 microsieverts (μSv) of radiological dose. But our CBCT only emits around 11 to 70 μSv of radiation, making it extremely low dose and extremely safe for patients. It is about equal to the daily exposure to radiation here on Earth. The International Commission on Radiological Protection (ICRP) recommends we keep non-occupation exposure levels less than 100,000 μSv per year.[9] We would have to take thousands of

---

9   ICRP, 2007. 2007 Recommendations of the International Commission on Radiological Protection (Users Edition), ICRP Publication 103 (Users Edition). Annual ICRP 37 (2-4).

images per year on a patient to have any discernible effects of exposure. Thus, it is safe to say that this technology is extremely beneficial with minimal risk.

PUTTING DOSE IN CONTEXT

Imaging Modality	Effective Dose µSv	Extra Days on Earth of Radiation Exposure
Routine X-rays at Dentist	171	21
Panoramic X-rays	19-24	2.5
CBCT at Dr. Klauer's	9-155	9

2,920 µSv Normal yearly radiation from living on Earth (8 µSv/day)

77 µSv i-CAT scan is a common scan we utilize and we routinely dose it less when indicated

CBCT also heightens the ability to identify osteoarthritis at early stages and accurately follow the condition during treatment. Osteoarthritis in the TM joint typically occurs because the patient has chronic inflammation that does not produce enough pain to warrant treatment or to justify going to see a provider, so the problem progresses. In the case of knees and hips, that explains how patients end up with artificial joints, but the TM joint is too complex to replace as readily as knees and hips, and there is a low success rate associated with TM joint surgery for treatment of TMD. We do have some very talented colleagues who perform TM joint replacements, but they agree that they are best utilized as a last resort or for developmental issues with the TM joints. So, the earlier we can diagnose and treat TMD, the better for the patient.

Once all the data from the tests is collected and reviewed, the exam concludes with a physical evaluation of the autonomic nervous system—those nerves that automatically control internal organs such as the heart, lungs, and stomach—using autonomic motor nerve reflex testing (AMNRT). As I mentioned before, these reflex tests developed and used by orthopedic surgeons allow me to identify the primary structural instability that is producing postural changes and posture avoidance in patients as it relates to their presenting symptoms. As Dr. John Beck states, in chronic pain situations, the location of pain is rarely the site of origin of the pain, thus making it prudent for us to find the origin of the patient's problem.

In his book *Finding the Source: Maximizing Your Results—With and Without Orthopaedic Surgery*, Dr. Victor Romano explains in detail how essential the autonomic motor nerve reflex testing is within his orthopedic practice. The true value of the reflex testing is that it shows us neurologically what the patient's primary pain problem is currently. Many of our patients have multiple layers of problems, and just because their chief complaint is facial pain doesn't mean the problem resides solely in or around the face. In his book, Dr. Romano goes on:

One study found that the more comorbidities, the more pain the patient may have—in other words, pain in one area may make them more susceptible to pain in another area.[10] For instance, the size of a rotator cuff tear may not correlate with the amount of pain a person is experiencing. They may also have pain coming from somewhere else in their body, and it's my job to find those comorbidities. If I can find and treat them, then the area where a patient is experiencing pain may improve without the need for surgery.[11]

RICK'S VICTORY

Rick's clinical examination revealed that he had capsulitis (inflammation) of the jaw joint and that his articular disc was dislocated. The TM joint condyle was flattened on top, indicating long-term forces in the joint complex. That was the source of his tension-type headaches, pain, and discomfort. The temples on either side of the head just behind the eyes and above the ears are the region of the temporalis muscles

---

10 Davis, Jessica, et. al, "Incidence and impact of pain conditions and comorbid illnesses," *Journal of Pain Research* 4 (2011): 331–345, accessed August 18, 2017 on U.S. Library of Medicine National Institutes of Health, https://www.ncbi.nlm.nih.gov/pmc/articles/PMC3215513/ quoted in Romano, Victor, *Finding the Source: Maximizing Your Results—With and Without Orthopaedic Surgery* (Charleston, S.C.: Advantage/Forbes Books, 2018).

11 Romano, Victor, *Finding the Source: Maximizing Your Results—With and Without Orthopaedic Surgery*, (Charleston, S.C.: Advantage/Forbes Books, 2018).

that helps to close the jaw. In Rick's case, the excessive firing of these muscles from his nighttime bruxism is what was contributing to his tension type headache. His motor nerve reflex testing illustrated that the orthopedic instability of his TM joint was his primary problem.

Since the nasal complex is in between the TM joints, we are able to capture the anatomical structures of the nose during examinations, placing us in a position of responsibility for making referrals for treatment when needed. Imaging of Rick's TM joint revealed a profound nasal obstruction that was preventing him from breathing properly through his nose. We noted a deviated septum and maxillary sinusitis (inflammation), which was consistent with his chronic symptoms of sinusitis, mouth breathing, and allergies. That led us to refer him to an ENT physician.

Given Rick's cardiac history of AFib and poor sleep, we also recommended a diagnostic sleep study to confirm or rule out OSA. Rick was non-obese, not even overweight, and had a low probability of OSA, but although we recommended an in-lab sleep test, his insurance dictated that he take a home sleep test.

Although he came in for evaluation of his sleep, we found that Rick's longstanding TM joint pain and difficulty breathing through his nose were likely culprits producing all his significant sleep symptoms. He agreed immediately, as the data collected was detailed, clear, and fit his clinical situation.

After all the testing, we determined that the best treatment for Rick was decompression orthotics to be worn day and night for twelve weeks. His diagnostic home sleep test came back within normal limits, and the sleep physician only recommended an in-lab sleep study if his symptoms did not improve during treatment, since home sleep tests can have false negative results. He wore the daytime orthotic on his mandible for twelve weeks, and the nighttime orthotic on his maxilla while he was sleeping. Together, the orthotics placed his jaw in a neutral position to allow for the TM joint complexes to heal. The orthotics were supplemented with home exercises and in-office physical therapy using photobiomodulation therapy (PBMT), also known as laser therapy, low-level laser therapy, and cold laser therapy. I will explain this in depth in Chapter 8.

We also felt that his cardiac condition could certainly improve, since the therapies helped to reestablish normal, functional nasal breathing and regulate his respiratory rhythm.

Just two weeks into treatment, Rick was already beginning to achieve his victory. He reported having fewer headaches, and the pain of those headaches had dropped from eight to two on a pain scale of zero to ten. He said he also fell asleep easier, slept better, and felt more rested in the morning—all of these improved by 50 to 70 percent or better within the first two weeks of treatment.

He still had some morning neck pain, so we administered trigger point injections into his trapezius (shoulder) muscles to help reduce some of his neck pain and spasms. Trigger point therapy is a great adjunct treatment we provide for many patients, giving immediate relief for specific situations. I will explain this treatment modality further in Chapter 8.

Rick was also happy to report that his heart palpitations ceased. In the past, a single glass of wine or a beer would cause his heart to flutter almost immediately. But after starting treatment, that didn't happen when he was at a summer cookout and indulged in a single beer. "For scientific purposes," he told me, he decided to try a second beer to test whether the improvement was real or just a fluke—happily, his heart didn't flutter even after beer number two.

Concurrently, his treatment also included chiropractic care from his existing doctor and correction of his deviated septum by an ENT physician.

After four weeks, Rick's symptoms were completely gone, and he had stopped taking his heart medications (under the direction of his cardiologist). At twelve weeks, we did a final evaluation on Rick to document all his improvements and to begin weaning him off his daytime orthotic. In medicine, we call this maximum medical improvement (MMI)—the point at which treatment reaches its peak improvement. Similar to treating a stress fracture, the twelve-week orthotic is designed to be worn while the jaw joint "heals," then it is removed rather than worn long term. Historically, patients with TMD were in orthotics for much longer periods (a year or more) and this was referred to as "Phase 1" treatment. After such a long period of use the teeth would shift so permanent changes to the dentition would need to be made. Patients would be transitioned into "Phase 2" treatment requiring new crowns or restorations throughout the mouth. It is a rare occasion that Phase 2 treatment occurs in our office, because we are comprehensively addressing the source of the problem and getting to the root cause. Phase 2 is an additional long-term treatment to the dentition needed to maintain a reduction of symptoms. Thankfully, we rarely need this in our office. Rick's before-and-after photos showed that his head was uprighted profoundly, his shoulders were situated back instead of forward, and his feet were no longer divergent. A cone beam computerized tomography (CBCT) scan taken at that point showed that his jaw joints were within normal limits, his nasal passages were far more open, and his sinus disease was completely resolved.

Rick's case illustrates how the TM joint can produce symptoms that appear to be unrelated. For Rick, what appeared to be a problem of sleep and headaches was actually a problem stemming from the jaw and the inability to breathe properly through his nose. That's why it's important to take a comprehensive approach to evaluating patients so that a proper diagnosis and effective treatment plan can be made. For Rick, treatment "changed everything," he said. "I sleep great now. I don't have pain. I feel so much better about not only my jaw and how my body feels, but I have so much more energy and I'm much, much happier."

Rick's situation explains how we must ensure a sound night's sleep void of any stimulation from pain and fragmentation from disordered breathing. His case also displays the body's habit to compensate for a problem by exhibiting symptoms that seem unrelated. In Rick's case, these symptoms would be his sleep problems and his headaches—things not caused by just surface-level factors, but by the issues embedded in his TM joints. Treatment proved that his cardiac issues (AFib) were caused by his chronic breathing issues and craniofacial pain. Once the body wasn't under distress, his cardiac issues self-resolved. It never ceases to amaze me that if we put the body the right environment, it will heal. The most gratifying part of what I do is reading testimonials from my patients, and I'm happy to say here that his victory was achieved!

> "After not sleeping well for an extended period of time, I longed to have a good night's sleep. Desperate for a solution, I sought care for my insomnia from Dr. Klauer, and informed him I had TMD. Uncertain of how they connected, but determined to sleep again, I followed all the treatment Dr. Klauer provided. In a short time, I was sleeping better, had fewer headaches, and even had decreased neck and back pain. At the completion of the treatment, I no longer had heart palpitations or arrhythmias I had been diagnosed with fifteen years earlier. Today, I have better posture, no jaw pain, and great sleep. The treatment and care has changed my life!" —Rick

In the next chapter, I will dive into the importance of sleep and how that is essential for patients to heal, recover, and go on living a great life.

CHAPTER 5
SLEEP SHOULD BE REJUVENATING

A person can go weeks without food, days without water, but only minutes without air.

When Ben came to see me for the first time, his chief complaint was debilitating fatigue. At age fifty-three, he was so tired that he didn't even have enough energy to leave the house. Ben was a heavy snorer who regularly had trouble falling asleep, woke up frequently during the night, and crawled out of bed groggy each morning. He never woke feeling refreshed. He also ground his teeth at night and had hypertension.

— VICTORY —

Ben's victory was to get some sleep and return to having a normal level of energy again.

Ben's victory was to get some sleep and return to having a normal level of energy again.

In Ben's clinical exam, we noted several signs and symptoms of obstructive sleep apnea (OSA) from the very beginning. He was unable to breathe through his nose due to chronic nasal congestion, so he primarily breathed with his mouth open—very unhealthy, as I've explained. He had a coating on his tongue, and his teeth were crooked and worn down from grinding at night.

As we explained these conditions to Ben, he became hopeful that they were the reasons for his fatigue. He was excited to undergo a sleep test and anxious to get the results so we could begin treatment.

SNORING
partial obstruction
of the airway

OSA
complete obstruction
of the airway

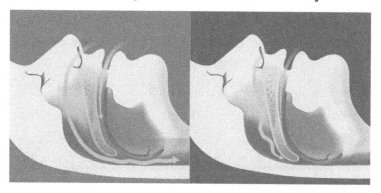

THE NEED FOR SLEEP

The truth is, no one really knows why we sleep. We know that all animals sleep and that sleep is essential for survival.

We also know that seventy million Americans suffer from a sleep problem, and that sleep deprivation will eventually lead to death. A study conducted at the University of Chicago on rats proved that after eleven days of hyperstimulation and no sleep, the rats died.[12] While there was no anatomical cause for death, all rats in the study showed debilitated appearance and abnormal growths on the body. The sleep deprivation literally killed them.

Numerous, complex tasks occur during sleep. But sleep disturbances—conditions that prevent or affect sleep—can rob the body of proper sleep, leading to a cascade of negative health consequences.

So, simply put, humans need sleep to survive, and the quality of sleep ultimately determines quality of life. Sleep gives the body a chance to rest, recover, and rejuvenate. It is the body's way of filling the tank back up with gas.

Children need to sleep more than adults because that is when their body is actually growing. Everyone knows the term "sleep like a baby." That's a sign of good health—a healthy child sleeps like a rock. But just like adults, children can have sleep disturbances. We all know children who don't sleep well—they typically have behavioral and developmental issues, because their brain and body aren't rejuvenating as intended each night. The correlation between ADHD and sleep disturbances in children is now clear and well docu-

---

12   Everson, CA, BM Bergmann, and A. Rechtschaffen, "Sleep deprivation in the rat: III. Total sleep deprivation," *Sleep*, vol. 12, no. 1(February 1989:13-21.

mented. There are numerous studies illustrating this that I'll go into depth about in Chapter 9, but let's not overlook the obvious fact that inadequate sleep will affect our physical and mental performance the following day—this is something we all have experienced at some time. If this is a nightly occurrence, then we will have a host of deeper medical issues. It is no different with adults; we need our sleep—sound sleep, uninterrupted sleep.

Sleep consists of two distinct states, REM (rapid eye movement) and non-REM. These two states alternate throughout the night in four or five cycles over the course of four to ten hours, depending on the individual. Seventy-five percent of sleep is non-REM, while REM sleep occupies typically the last quarter or third of the night.

Non-REM sleep is the state of sleep responsible for physical restoration and is characterized by what are known as delta waves, which are slow brain waves. In adults, 90 percent of repair of damaged tissue occurs during sleep. Non-REM is the greatest portion of sleep in children, but the length of time a person spends in non-REM decreases from ages fifty to sixty-five. By age sixty-five, non-REM sleep can be absent.[13]

REM sleep typically accounts for 25 percent of a night's sleep. REM is responsible for improving learning, memory attention, and the ability to focus throughout the day. That is why staying up late to cram for a test may not be a good

---

13 Meir Kryger, Thomas Roth, and William Dement, *Principles and Practice of Sleep Medicine*, 5th ed. (Philadelphia: Saunders, 2010).

idea, because it ultimately causes a lack of REM sleep—meaning the new material just read won't be retained as well, if at all. You may remember it for tomorrows test but when you need that information weeks later it may not be recalled. REM sleep is characterized by reduced muscle activity and paralysis, which can predispose the airway to further collapse, worsening any sleep breathing disorders (SBDs) or resulting in a REM-dependent SBD.

CAUSES AND SYMPTOMS

What exactly are SBD and OSA? SBD occurs when a person stops breathing, either partially or completely, many times throughout the night. That can result in daytime sleepiness or fatigue that often reduces quality of life and inability to function throughout the day.

There are three types of SBD: snoring, upper airway resistance syndrome (UARS), and OSA. OSA is the most common form of SBD. It is associated with many negative health consequences, including chronic diseases and even death.

While we can't say for certain what one thing causes OSA, there are many predisposing factors contributing to this debilitating disease.

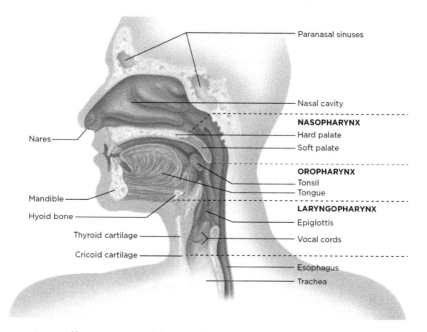

Paranasal sinuses

Nasal cavity

NASOPHARYNX
Hard palate
Soft palate

Nares

OROPHARYNX
Tonsil
Tongue

Mandible

LARYNGOPHARYNX
Hyoid bone
Epiglottis

Thyroid cartilage
Vocal cords

Cricoid cartilage

Esophagus
Trachea

A small airway. Problems of the oral airway include a small opening anatomically, which increases the chances of the airway collapsing during sleep. The narrower a tube, the greater the likelihood of collapse.

Improper maxilla and mandible development. Improper development of the maxilla and mandible can also predispose an individual to obstruction of the airway. If the maxilla and mandible aren't fully developed forward and wide, it will reduce the dimensions of the airway. Again, this increases the chances of collapse.

Crooked teeth. Malocclusion (crooked teeth) indicate that there is inadequate space for the tongue inside the mouth.

The tongue ultimately determines how teeth are situated in the mouth, and malocclusion indicates that the tongue—a huge muscle—has limited room. When there's not enough room, the tongue can obstruct the airway. The orthodontic textbook *Contemporary Orthodontics* states, "Respiratory patterns are the primary determinant of the position of the head, jaw, and teeth."[14] That helps us understand the relationship between orthopedic development of the face and breathing. It doesn't mean, however, that someone with straight teeth can't have obstructive breathing—only that the likelihood increases with malocclusion.

Swollen airway tissues. Tonsils and adenoids are lymphatic tissue that rest in the back of the throat and nasal cavity. If these are swollen, they will also take up space within the airway and cause breathing problems.

Overweight. Obesity causes increased fat deposition in the soft-tissue passages of the airway and decreased muscle tone, making it more difficult to breathe and increasing the chances of an airway collapse at night.

Pregnancy. Pregnancy can cause increased inflammation and increased weight on the mother's diaphragm, leading to a higher chance of experiencing a collapse of the airway. That can lead to decreased oxygen levels (hypoxia) in the mother,

---

14   Proffit, William, Henry Fields, and David Sarver, *Contemporary Orthodontics* (St. Louis, Missouri: Mosby Elsevier, 2007).

which is not good for the baby and can increase the chances of preeclampsia during pregnancy.

Nasal obstructions. Nasal airway problems can also cause airway obstruction. These include a deviated septum (a crooked nasal bone), bone spurs in the nose, swollen nasal tissue, chronic sinus congestion, and allergies. These can decrease the flow of air through the nasal passages, decreasing the amount of oxygen getting to the lungs. When the muscles relax during sleep, that decreased airflow can cause OSA. A great study by Dr. M.F. Fitzpatrick and others illustrated that upper airway resistance during sleep and propensity to OSA are significantly lower while breathing nasally than while breathing orally. As I mentioned earlier in the book, nasal breathing is normal breathing. It is abnormal to routinely breathe through the mouth.[15]

COMMON SYMPTOMS OF SBD

There are several common symptoms of SBD and OSA. Historically, snoring and jerking awake gasping for breath are believed to be the only signs and symptoms of OSA. Although they are common, not everyone with SBD has those two symptoms. Here is what we commonly see in the new patients we welcome to our practice daily.

---

15   Fitzpatrick, M.F. et al., "Effect of nasal or oral breathing route on upper airway resistance during sleep," *European Respiratory Journal* 22 (2003): 827-832.

- ☐ Nerve pain
- ☐ Acid indigestion
- ☐ Kicking or jerking leg repeatedly
- ☐ Swelling in ankles or feet
- ☐ Morning hoarseness in voice
- ☐ Dry mouth upon waking
- ☐ Fatigue
- ☐ Difficulty falling asleep
- ☐ Frequent tossing and turning
- ☐ Repeated awakening
- ☐ Nighttime urination
- ☐ Significant daytime drowsiness
- ☐ Frequent heavy snoring
- ☐ Feeling unrefreshed in the morning
- ☐ Affecting sleep of others
- ☐ Gasping upon waking
- ☐ Told that "I stop breathing" during sleep
- ☐ Nighttime choking spells
- ☐ Morning headaches
- ☐ Night sweats
- ☐ Vivid dreaming
- ☐ Unable to tolerate CPAP
- ☐ Teeth grinding
- ☐ Teeth crowding

Another hallmark sign of OSA is insomnia. Insomnia is described as the inability to fall asleep or the drive to stay awake. Oftentimes, people with insomnia think their problem is just that they can't fall asleep. They don't realize that it may have something to do with the brain's drive to keep them awake. It is plausible to surmise that if the brain knows that you're going to start suffocating as soon as you fall asleep, it is going to work to keep you awake as long as possible, because it is conditioned to believe that on the other side of that suffocating sleep is death (not breathing, that is).

And sleep medications, it turns out, are really not a viable long-term solution for most insomnia patients. A recent study by the Mayo Clinic and the Human Health Institute investigated drug failure in 1,210 chronic insomnia patients, meaning that over-the-counter and doctor-supervised prescription drugs had failed to treat their insomnia. Once patients failed to get results with their medications sleep studies were performed on all the patients. The results of the study were astounding: 91 percent of the subjects suffered from undiagnosed OSA, a critical factor likely to be aggravating their insomnia.[16]

Waking up to use the restroom at night is also a common symptom of SBD. There are two reasons this might occur. One is that OSA places more pressure on the heart, resulting in an increased workload that increases the amount of fluid

---

16   "Insomniacs Failing Drugs Suffer from Sleep Apnea," Yahoo Finance, September 15, 2014, accessed October 19, 2017, https://finance. yahoo.com/news/insomniacs-failing-drugs-suffer-sleep-130000210. html.

going to the kidneys. That increases urine production during sleep, making a person wake up to void more often. The other reason is that a hormone (vasopressin, aka the antidiuretic hormone) produced during sleep helps retain fluid in the periphery, outside the bladder, during sleep, so the person doesn't have to wake up to void. When a person doesn't get to the appropriate stages of sleep, that hormone is not being produced, leaving the bladder to fill up and cause a need to urinate more frequently. In adults, that means getting up frequently at night to use the restroom. In children, it often means wetting the bed (nocturnal enuresis).

DEBILITATING HEALTH ISSUES

The aforementioned symptoms are often debilitating enough on their own, but when coupled with the long-term effects of OSA, the results can be devastating. OSA has been shown to lead to high blood pressure, heart disease, stroke, type II diabetes, metabolic syndrome, and liver problems. Aside from the health risks, patients often face declining job performance and jeopardized relationships due to the pain and fatigue they endure throughout the day.

Current literature supports the relationship between TMD and OSA. Patients diagnosed with TMD have an increased prevalence of OSA; patients diagnosed with OSA have an increased prevalence of TMD. My mentor, Dr. Olmos, writes of research on two separate studies of 2,604 and 1,716 patients:

*Two studies tested the hypothesis that OSA signs and symptoms were associated with TMD. ... Both studies supported a significant relationship between OSA symptoms and TMD with prospective cohort evidence finding that **OSA symptoms preceded first-onset of TMD**: patients with two or more signs and/or symptoms of OSA had a 73 percent greater incidence of first onset TMD.*[17]

OSA can also lead to TMD because clenching and grinding is felt to be a response to the stimulus of a collapsing or constricted airway. Over time, that repetitive trauma can cause inflammation and damage to the TM joint.

Dr. David Gozal of the University of Chicago has also linked untreated OSA to increased incidence and recurrence of cancer, due in part to the intermittent hypoxia (deficiency in the amount of oxygen reaching tissues) combined with the fragmented sleep that comes with OSA. He suggests that OSA promotes changes that can cause malignant tumors to transform and expand, which can lead to an increased probability of accelerated tumor growth and proliferation.[18]

---

17 Olmos, Steven, "Comorbidities of chronic facial pain and obstructive sleep apnea," *Current Opinion in Pulmonary Medicine* 22, no. 6 (November 2016): 570–575.

18 Gozal, David, Ramon Farré, and F. Javier Nieto, "Putative Links Between Sleep Apnea and Cancer," *Chest*, vol. 148, no. 5(November 2015):1140-1147, accessed February 15, 2018 on U.S. Library of Medicine National Institutes of Health, https://www.ncbi.nlm.nih.gov/pmc/articles/PMC4631033.

Hypoxia *is the deficiency in the amount of oxygen reaching tissues.* **Hypoxemia** *is the deficiency of oxygen concentration in the blood.*

Many of the debilitating health issues of untreated OSA stem from the increase in brain arousals and the decrease in oxygen levels. Hypoxemia (abnormally low oxygen concentration in the blood), is extremely damaging to the body's cells and causes destruction. Remember, nothing trumps breathing. OSA is damaging because the moment the brain experiences deprivation of air, it sends an arousal signal—which is essentially a shot of adrenaline (epinephrine) and cortisol—to stimulate the body to wake up and resume breathing. That is done repeatedly throughout the night and is extremely damaging to the body. Some experts say that OSA should stand for "obstructive sleep arousals" rather than apnea because the arousals damage the body and cause increased inflammation, which results in cellular destruction.

Decreased oxygen levels are also detrimental to health. Bodily tissues and organs need oxygen for survival. When breathing stops, oxygen saturation levels go down, depriving the tissues of oxygen. That leads to organ damage and tissue necrosis, or even death.

Hormone creation is also disrupted when sleep is constantly interrupted. The endocrine system has complex responses to sleep. The endocrine system is a collection of glands that secrete hormones into the circulatory system that are then carried to other organs. During sleep, the secretion of some hormones (growth, prolactin, and luteinizing hormones) increases, while the secretion of other hormones (thyroid-stimulating hormones and cortisol) is inhibited.

Some hormones are tied to a specific stage of sleep. Growth hormone, for instance, is secreted during the first few hours of sleep and is generally released during slow-wave sleep—the delta-wave sleep I mentioned earlier. Delta sleep is the deep sleep in which the body is physically restored and growth actually occurs.

Cortisol—the stress hormone—is tied to the circadian rhythm (the sleep/wake cycle). Regardless of how well someone sleeps, cortisol is released during the day and peaks late in the afternoon. But when a breathing event wakes a person up at night, cortisol is secreted to keep the person awake so that they can resume breathing. That leads to an inordinate amount of cortisol being secreted at night, promoting wakefulness and ultimately raising stress levels. Remember that Mayo Clinic study mentioned earlier? Those patients suffered from insomnia and could not fall asleep. It is likely that their cortisol levels were extremely elevated due to their OSA.

Hormones from the pituitary gland have secretion levels intimately related to the sleep pattern. Production of melatonin—the sleep hormone—is also disrupted in patients with sleep disorders. Melatonin is released in the dark and is suppressed by light—as it starts to get dark outside, melatonin is secreted to promote sleep. Growth hormone (vital in adults for tissue repair and in children for growth) and prolactin both peak at the onset of sleep. Testosterone secretion is elevated at the beginning of sleep and continues to increase through the night. Most hormones peak during non-REM sleep. Here again, sleep fragmentation and hypoxia from OSA cause abnormalities in hormone production and a rise in adrenaline.

Lastly, diabetes is a specific disease that affects the endocrine system's ability to produce the hormone insulin, and it is in turn affected by sleep. Adults who get less than five hours of sleep at night are more likely to have diabetes, compared to those who sleep seven to eight hours per night. Interestingly, people who sleep more than nine hours per night also have increased rates of diabetes. Patients suffering from OSA have increased glucose levels, and the more severe the OSA, the higher the glucose levels.[19] Thus, we know Type 2 Diabetes (non-insulin dependent diabetes) is a risk factor for OSA, and having OSA will increase the likelihood of developing OSA. In Type 2 Diabetes your body is resisting the effects of insulin or doesn't produce enough insulin to maintain your glucose levels. Unfortunately, as our diets get worse and worse, the rate of Type 2 Diabetes get higher and higher.

---

19   Pamidi, Sushmita, Renee Aronsohn, and Esra Tasali, "Obstructive Sleep Apnea: Role in the Rick and Severity of Diabetes," *Best Practice & Research Clinical Endocrinology & Metabolism* 24, no. 5 (October 2, 2010): 703-715, accessed February 19, 2018 on U.S. Library of Medicine National Institutes of Health, *https://www.ncbi.nlm.nih.gov/pmc/articles/PMC2994098.*

Whatever the cause, fragmented sleep has a direct influence on pain thresholds, cognitive function, anxiety and depression, and other issues, both chronic and debilitating.

IDENTIFYING AND DIAGNOSING OSA

While a sleep study is always needed to confirm whether OSA is at play or not, evaluation of the anatomical structures associated with OSA is also incredibly important. To do that, we use advanced imaging technology and diagnostic tools to accurately identify potential areas of concern and create an optimal treatment plan.

There are often structural risk factors seen during an evaluation that allow us to identify that a patient might have SBD or OSA. Again, oral airway problems, mouth breathing, and bruxism all give insight as to what might be happening at night during sleep.

Facial development issues—a high palate, narrow dental arch, malocclusion (crooked teeth), excessive overjet (upper teeth jutting outward)—all may indicate OSA. The palate (roof of the mouth) is made up of two bones, connected by a suture, that are extremely malleable in children. The forces of breast-feeding and the movement of the tongue stimulate optimal growth of the palate. Proper nasal breathing coupled with breast-feeding and normal swallow leads to ideal facial development.

Oftentimes we see that patients who grew up without breast-feeding breathe through their mouths and have less-than-ideal facial development. These craniofacial variations have proven to be risk indicators and predictive of SBD. These are findings that can only be revealed with a detailed medical history during the evaluation to discuss signs, symptoms, and risk factors of OSA.

Scalloped tongue is also predictive of OSA; it's a 70 percent indicator, according to ENT physician literature.[20] Scalloped tongue is identified by crenations, or notches, along the sides of the tongue caused by the tongue pushing up against the teeth all night long.

In evaluating patients with sleep disturbances and failure to improve their sleep with other techniques and treatment, it is essential to order a diagnostic sleep study. Right now, a sleep test diagnosed by a sleep physician is the only way to confirm or rule out SBD. We cannot rely on the observations of a bed partner. Hopefully the bed partner is busy sleeping soundly themselves. Also, I often tell patients that while snoring is a hallmark sign of OSA, the sound of not breathing is silence—so if someone is not breathing intermittently, there is really nothing to hear.

A diagnostic sleep study can determine whether SBD is present, and if so, the severity of the disorder. Physicians, physician's assistants, dentists, chiropractors, nurses, and

---

20 Weiss, TM, S. Atanasov, and K.H. Calhoun, "The association of tongue scalloping with obstructive sleep apnea and related sleep pathology," *Otolaryngology-Head and Neck Surgery* 133, no. 6 (December 2005): 966–71, accessed February 19, 2018 on U.S. Library of Medicine National Institutes of Health, https://www.ncbi.nlm.nih.gov/pubmed/16360522.

primary care doctors can order diagnostic sleep studies—depending on the hospital system, insurance, and the state. However, only a sleep physician can review the sleep test and provide the actual diagnosis. It's kind of like a radiologist reading a hospital CT scan. Tests may be performed by a radiology tech, but the patient never really meets the radiologist who reads the results of the tests and makes a diagnosis that is delivered to the treating physician. While we prefer the patient to meet face-to-face with a sleep physician, it is not always possible, as there are not enough sleep physicians to feasibly see all the patients diagnosed with SBD.

There are basically two types of sleep tests: home tests and in-lab tests. Home tests are commonly referred to as HSTs (home sleep tests) or out-of-center sleep studies. Home tests are done in the confines of the patient's home and include a monitoring/recording unit along with a strap that wraps around the chest, a probe worn on the finger, and a cannula worn by the nose. The devices record breathing activity, body movement and position, oxygen levels, and respiratory effort throughout the night. That information is then scored and reviewed by a registered polysomnographic technologist (RPGST) and a sleep physician to render a diagnosis.

An in-lab sleep test (polysomnography/polysomnogram) uses more detailed equipment to measure brainwave activity (electroencephalography, or EEG). This test is actively monitored throughout the night by a sleep technician. This information is then similarly scored and reviewing by an RPGST and a sleep physician to render a diagnosis.

Every day, I explain the sleep tests like this: Home sleep tests are more accurate sleep but less accurate data. In-lab sleep tests are more accurate data but less accurate sleep. Generally speaking, patients sleep better at home and in their own beds. However, home sleep tests can have false negatives, inaccurately identifying someone as being "normal." This is where a good clinical history and follow-up is needed to order subsequent testing as needed. The trend is certainly going toward more home testing, as the technology is rapidly improving and if a home test doesn't show us the results needed, an in-lab test can always be ordered.

Regardless of which study is used, the results of the study are reported as a score referred to as the respiratory disturbance index (RDI), the apnea-hypopnea index (AHI), or the respiratory event index (REI). These terms are relatively synonymous, and it depends on the sleep lab and the sleep physician as to which term is used. RDI encompasses RERA (respiratory effort-related arousal), while AHI and REI are just inclusive of apneas and hypopneas. The events are totaled and divided by the hours of sleep, which results in an index.

THREE MAIN SCORING CRITERIA WITH DIAGNOSTIC SLEEP TESTS.

Apnea – a cessation of breathing for at least ten seconds (at least a 90 percent reduction in airflow from baseline breathing) associated with a 3 percent reduction of blood oxygen saturation levels, resulting in an arousal to resume normal breathing.

Hypopnea – a 30 percent reduction of airflow for at least ten seconds associated with a 3 percent reduction in blood oxygen saturation levels, resulting in an arousal.

RERA – (respiratory effort-related arousal) characterized by obstructive upper airway airflow reduction associated with increased respiratory effort that resolves with the appearance of arousals.

Basically, what these indexes report is how many times per hour of sleep the brain is awakened due to a respiratory event or a break in breathing. OSA is defined as a cessation of breathing during sleep for at least ten seconds. A score of normal is equal to less than five events per hour of sleep, while higher scores are classified as shown in the following table.

APNEA-HYPOPNEA INDEX (AHI)

SEVERITY	AHI PER HOUR	
	Adults	Children
Mild	5-15	1-5
Moderate	16-30	6-10
Severe	>30	>10

BEN'S VICTORY

When Ben's sleep study results were returned, it showed severe sleep apnea. At 36.9 breathing events per hour of sleep, he was waking about once every two minutes. Think about how that kind of fragmented sleep would affect a person the following day. What's interesting is that Ben wasn't aware that he was waking up once every two minutes. He was so tired and exhausted that his brain basically would wake up just enough to resume breathing, and then he would fall back asleep.

At first, Ben needed care from our trusted referral partners in order to adequately treat his severe sleep apnea. He was originally started on a continuous positive airway pressure (CPAP) machine, which supplied him with air through a hose and a mask that he wore over his nose and mouth at night while he slept. Ben tried the CPAP diligently for weeks, but ultimately, he could not tolerate it, so under the order of his sleep physician, we customized an oral appliance for him to wear nightly. Ben's specific appliance was designed to prevent the retrusion of his mandible while sleeping. By preventing his mandible from falling back, the appliance holds his tongue, soft palate, and associated tissue slightly forward and prevents the collapse of his airway.

After the very first night of sleep, Ben reported that he woke up feeling amazing. He slept soundly through the night and did not wake up fatigued. And his wife reported that his snoring had stopped. Now, everyone doesn't have such quick results, but our ultimate goal is to achieve their victory.

In the months following, we continued to see Ben to adjust his appliance and ensure that we stayed on track for properly treating his OSA. During that time, he also needed treatment for chronic nasal congestion by an ENT physician.

Today, I'm happy to report that Ben's OSA is being adequately controlled, as validated by a follow-up sleep study with his appliance in place. His breathing events have dropped below five per hour, which is well within the normal and acceptable range for an individual. Ben says his treatment improved life for him and everyone around him. As Ben describes it, he went from a zombie-like existence to being able to walk miles every day—that's rewarding to hear from a patient.

"There's no more snoring, thank God, and [I'm] breathing easier—everything in that respect has just made my life much better. It's better for me, for my wife, for my children. ... I feel healthier. And I was in a pretty bad state, so if it can work for me, it can certainly work for others who don't have the condition nearly as bad as I did."

Sometimes, I think it would be great if patients came to us with just one problem, whether that's just facial pain or only a problem sleeping. But unfortunately, that's not the case. Often patients are plagued with both pain and sleep problems, which mandates that we evaluate their chronic facial pain along with their chronic sleep disturbances, and often we've found that chronic sleep disturbances and facial pain cannot be separated. They're intimately related, and we have to sift through the patient's clinical history to determine the primary cause of the problem.

That often leads to a "chicken and egg" conundrum: Which came first? Did the facial pain aggravate the chronic sleep problem or did the chronic sleep and breathing problem aggravate the patient's chronic facial pain? In the next chapter, I will discuss this conundrum and explain which came first.

CHAPTER 6
TMD AND SLEEP APNEA— THE "WHICH CAME FIRST?" CONUNDRUM

There is an inseparable truth about TMD and SBD.

Sixty-eight-year-old Donna was referred to us by an endodontist (a root canal specialist) because she had a lot of jaw pain when chewing. She had gone to the endodontist because she thought her jaw pain was coming from a tooth, but when he could not find anything wrong, he asked us to evaluate her. In addition to the jaw pain, Donna also had numerous other symptoms: jaw joint noises, sore jaw upon waking, neck pain, sinus congestion, dizziness, GERD, difficulty falling asleep, tossing and turning all night, fatigue, feeling unrefreshed in the morning, tinnitus (ringing in the ear), ear stuffiness, and ear congestion.

Donna's victory was to eliminate her jaw and tooth pain, which she said had plagued her for as long as she could remember. Donna had actually experienced one jaw issue or another since she was a teenager, including pain, clicking and popping, and grinding of teeth during the night—all on the left side of her face. She had seen four different doctors for evaluation and treatment of her TMD problems, and over the years she'd had ten different types of appliances made for her. Hard, soft, big, small, removable, permanent, part time, full time—she had worn just about every style or type of appliance out there. She felt that using so many treatments to chase her jaw pain had finally made it impossible for her to even bite properly.

—— VICTORY ——

Donna's victory was to eliminate her jaw and tooth pain, which she said had plagued her for as long as she could remember.

Her most recent treatment had been four years earlier with a dentist who ultimately dismissed her after growing frustrated with being unable to relieve her pain. Understandably, Donna had grown frustrated as well with the inability of so many providers to resolve her problems.

She finally resorted to taking Benadryl nightly to fall asleep, but she always awoke with a headache. She was emphatic that her sleep was not an issue and that it was normal for her not to sleep well, a statement we hear daily at our office.

In addition to the treatments for her jaw pain, Donna had been treated for GERD, anxiety, arthritis, hypothyroidism, skin cancer, cold hands and feet, muscle aches and cramps, sinusitis, and chronic temporal headaches on the left side. She had also already undergone a tonsillectomy, nasal surgery, sinus surgery, microdiscectomy on her neck, and an inner ear perfusion.

After careful review of Donna's medical history and her current symptoms, we explained that we needed to do a comprehensive evaluation that included imaging of the TM joints. Given her history and symptoms, it was evident that she was suffering from TMD, since she had all the classic symptoms: bruxism, clicking and popping of the jaw, facial pain, jaw pain, ear pain, tinnitus, dizziness, headaches, and so on—but then again, this was nothing she didn't already know.

I went on to explain to her that I thought there was more going on than just TMD. After all, if it was solely TMD and nothing more, why was she in our office after all those treatments from other providers? Clearly the root cause of her problem had yet to be identified.

THERE IS A CONNECTION

Explaining to a patient who clearly has TMD that something else is at the root of their problems is a crucial point in the relationship. I have to be extremely careful to ensure the patient knows I have listened to them and heard that their chief complaint is pain and not necessarily sleep problems, but that the two are often intimately related. I have to move cautiously when I present a way of looking at things that has never been proposed—in Donna's case, by multiple providers over a forty-year period. The question I get every single day is: "Why didn't anyone tell me this before now?" *And that's precisely why I wrote this book!*

At that point in the relationship with Donna, I asked if she'd be willing to do me a favor if I accepted her as a patient and completed a comprehensive exam and imaging of her TM joints. Of course, she wanted to know what the favor was. Now, sometimes, I'm a bit blunt or forward with patients, but I also try to be very empathetic and respectful, understanding that they have been through a great deal. In regard to the favor, I told Donna, "As I review your medical history, a lot of things stand out to me about your sleep: bruxism, frequent waking, difficulty falling asleep, feeling unrefreshed in the morning, morning headaches, sore jaw upon waking, fatigue, morning hoarseness in your voice, Benadryl every night needed to sleep, nighttime GERD, and waking with anxiety. With so many symptoms, I think it would be foolish of us not to evaluate your sleep as we evaluate your TMD. So with that, will you agree to complete a one-night sleep test so that we can help you achieve your victory?"

As is the case with many patients, Donna resisted, insisting that sleep had nothing to do with her problems.

"I've always been a bad sleeper," she said, to which I politely replied, "Precisely. You've always had TMD, too."

She got a good chuckle out of my quick reply and responded with "Well, if my sleep was a problem, wouldn't someone else have already evaluated that?"

I reminded her that she asked to be evaluated by me, and that's what I was doing. "Look," I said. "If you have a problem sleeping, what better way to find out than to undergo a sleep test? You sleep every night anyway—or at least you try to. So let's simply evaluate you one night to see what's happening." I went on to explain the inseparable connection between TMD and sleep breathing disorder (SBD). Finally, Donna agreed to the sleep test and we proceeded with our evaluation and imaging.

Our clinical findings illustrated that anatomically, Donna's TM joints were relatively within normal limits. She did have profound muscular pain and discomfort, which was producing a lot of her symptoms, but she had no osteoarthritis and no permanent locking of the TM joint or deterioration of the associated structures. There was no inherent damage to her TM joints—none. Basically, she did not have a primary TMD problem, yet she had been treated like a patient with a primary TMD problem. What I'm saying is that her TM joints were not the problem. I will repeat that again; her TM joints were not the problem. They were a symptom of a greater problem. That is likely why her symptoms hadn't improved through multiple treatments—the wrong thing was being treated.

The most significant clinical findings in the exam were her abnormal nasal and sinus passages, along with a significantly narrow airway. I explained to Donna that we could certainly help reduce her muscular pain and headaches, but I thought that could only be accomplished by eventually treating her suspected obstructive sleep apnea (OSA).

Donna proceeded with a home sleep test, completed by a sleep physician, and the results shocked her. The test showed that she basically stopped breathing 29.7 times per hour. So, nearly thirty times an hour, her brain was sending a signal to her body to resume breathing adequately. Thirty times an hour, her breathing was getting blocked or so slowed that her oxygen levels dropped to the point of potentially damaging her tissues. Thirty times an hour, her body was getting a shock of adrenaline to wake her up and start breathing again. Did I mention that the test showed us she was suffocating thirty times per hour and she had no clue?

We coupled the diagnostic testing results with our clinical evaluation and developed a great game plan for achieving Donna's victory of eliminating her jaw and tooth pain, while also tremendously improving things she didn't even know could be improved. Her tooth pain that brought her to the endodontist was merely referred pain from her bruxism associated with undiagnosed OSA—how's that for a connection?

The sleep physician proposed treating her OSA with an FDA-approved oral appliance given her profound history of bruxism and need to protect her dentition and reduce her facial pain. The multipurpose appliance was designed to address her collapsing oral structures, leading to her OSA, while also keeping her TM joints in an orthopedically stable position and decreasing her muscular activity. That would treat all her chief complaints, as well as the root origin of her problem. That was really exciting for us.

Before Oral Appliance　　　With Oral Appliance

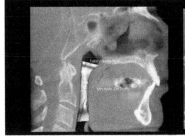 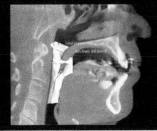

Total Volume: 17.4 cc　　　Total Volume: 31.9 cc
Min Area: 209.7mm2　　　Min Area: 405.5mm2

TIME TO GET A BIT TECHNICAL

My goal in this book has been not to get too technical, but at this point, I feel you're ready for some details about the intimate relationship between OSA and TMD—as in Donna's case.

That's the ultimate question: Which came first, the chicken or the egg? Or, as it applies to this discussion, which came first, TMD or OSA? The quick answer is that breathing trumps pain. Breathing and adequate sleep are essential for existence, and that cannot be refuted. Taking that one step further: functional, healthy breathing should be primarily through the nose as nature intended.

If breathing trumps all, and the goal is to find the origin of the problem, then let's start by looking at how OSA came into existence and why people develop it.

The human airway begins at the tip of the nose and includes the passages through the nose, through the back of the mouth, and down to the epiglottis, which is the structure that helps facilitate food going into the stomach and air going into the lungs. During swallowing, the epiglottis closes over the trachea (passage tube to lungs) to prevent aspiration of food into the lungs, ensuring that liquids or foods go down the esophagus (passage tube to stomach) to the stomach.

Sleep apnea was first discovered in 1965. Drs. Christian Guilleminault and William Dement developed the first diagnostic criteria for OSA. As a side note, I had the pleasure of lecturing with Dr. Guilleminault at one of our most recent academy meetings. It was an honor and privilege to be alongside the "Father of Sleep."

These two men are the pioneers in sleep. They discovered the different stages of sleep and really brought an understanding to the phenomenon that is studied today. Prior to 1965, sleep apnea was called Pickwickian syndrome, after a character who falls asleep standing up in Charles Dickens's first novel, *The Pickwick Papers*. Doctors thought this dysfunction was limited to obese patients, but later determined that although obesity increases the chance of OSA, it is not the sole cause. Non-obese patients and underweight patients can and do have OSA. We see it every day in our practice; you don't have to be overweight to snore and have OSA.

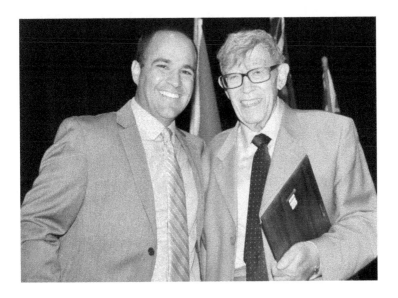

OSA began to be understood as a complex medical condition caused by the position of the tongue and the tissues of the throat. It was given the name "apnea," which is the Greek word for breathless. In understanding more about apnea, it was discovered that besides English bulldogs and pugs, humans are the only animals to experience sleep apnea. It is purely a result of evolution and the human ability to walk upright and speak combined with the decreasing dimensions of the face, specifically the nose and mouth—a narrow nose means a narrow mouth. After all, as I mentioned earlier, the top of the mouth is the bottom of the nose.

Consider the evolution of man: A Neanderthal's jawbones were much larger and stronger than those of humans today, providing for extra room in the mouth. Neanderthals never had impacted wisdom teeth (third molars). Homo sapiens differed from this by developing a flatter face and a tongue that descends deeper into the throat. With these changes and evolutions, humans were able to start making simple grunts, which then developed into language. The vocal chords and muscles of the throat allow us to phonate. But like all muscles, these relax and decrease in muscle tone during sleep.

Today's smaller mouth complicates the acts of eating, breathing, and drinking. Moving forward through evolution, the pushed-back faces and narrow dental arches that humans developed predisposed them to have airways that can collapse and tissues that relax when sleep sets in.

So it is now understood that the evolution of the human face, the narrower jaws, and the ability to speak is what predisposed humans to the chance of developing SBD. While obesity is a risk factor, as stated before, it is not the end-all and be-all, and narrower jaws and pushed-back faces are common risk indicators that someone may develop OSA. In fact, patients of Asian descent have greater likelihood of SBD due to their facial structures, specifically midface deficiencies.[21]

A couple of studies illustrate the importance of breathing through the nose and what may happen without adequately breathing through the nose as a person grows and develops. Dr. Egil Harvold conducted an experiment on growing rhesus monkeys that showed that if the nasal passages were blocked, facial development was altered, teeth became more crooked,

---

21 Aibek E. Mirrakhimov, Talant Sooronbaev, and Erkin M. Mirrakhimov, "Prevalence of obstructive sleep apnea in Asian adults: a systematic review of the literature," *BMC Pulm Med* 13, no. 10 (February 2013), https://doi.org/ 10.1186/1471-2466-13-10

dental arches became narrower, and the mandible did not develop as far forward. Dr. Harvold blocked the noses and observed the changes quickly. As he removed the blockage the growing monkeys started to return towards the normal appearance. This study simply illustrates the importance of breathing through the nose and how that helps develop craniofacial structures to their full dimension.[22]

Furthermore, the medical textbook *Contemporary Orthodontics* illustrates that respiratory patterns dictate facial development:

> "Respiratory needs are the primary determinant of the posture of the jaws and the tongue (and the head itself, to a lesser extent). Therefore, it seems entirely reasonable that an altered respiratory pattern, such as breathing through the mouth rather than the nose, could change the posture of the head, jaw, and tongue. ... In order to breathe through the mouth, it is necessary to lower the mandible and tongue and extend (tip back) the head. If these postural changes were maintained, face height would increase, and posterior teeth would super-erupt..."[23]

The result would be teeth that aren't straight.

---

22 Harvold, Egil, et al., "Primate experiments on oral respiration," *American Journal of Orthodontics* 70, no. 4 (April 1981): 359-72.

23 Proffit, William, Henry Fields, and David Sarver, *Contemporary Orthodontics* (St. Louis, Missouri: Mosby Elsevier, 2007), 154.

As people grow into adulthood, nasal breathing is paramount to ensuring that OSA doesn't develop. Dr. Guilleminault strongly believes that OSA is preventable in many people if we accurately identify those individuals early in life. In looking at Donna's medical history, it was obvious that she had many symptoms that pointed to her developing OSA.

Dr. Olmos has eloquently explained that there is an established relationship between OSA and TMD and presented evidence that they are bidirectional.

> There is an increased prevalence of TMD in patients diagnosed with OSA. There is an increased prevalence of OSA in patients diagnosed with TMD. Two studies tested the hypothesis that OSA signs and symptoms were associated with TMD. ... Both studies supported the significant association between OSA symptoms and TMD, with prospective cohort evidence finding that OSA symptoms precede first-onset of TMD: patients with two or more signs and/or symptoms of OSA had a 73% greater incidence of first-onset TMD.[24]

Dr. Olmos's article cites two studies that looked at more than 4,300 individuals combined and found that breathing symptoms preceded TMD and that breathing problems

---

24 Olmos, Steven, "Comorbidities of chronic facial pain and obstructive sleep apnea," *Current Opinion in Pulmonary Medicine* 22, no. 6 (November 2016): 570-575.

increase the risk of developing TMD.[25] That further supports the notion that breathing trumps pain. Dr. Olmos and others also found an association between TM joint locking, headaches, and daytime sleepiness,[26] illustrating that patients with TMD symptoms are commonly suffering from sleep problems, and a great deal of these TMD problems are potentially undiagnosed SBD problems too.

Look at the priority of life: The human body can suffer pain. It can walk through pain. But it can't suffer through an inability to breathe. The body will compensate by changing the position of the neck and tongue to ventilate as best it can. Without breath, death is imminent, so the body makes trade-offs to continue breathing at whatever cost, and that results in all the problems I've been talking about in this book—all the problems that Donna was having.

Still, it takes a diagnostic workup to prove to patients—and to ourselves—that their breathing and sleep may be the root of their problems. If so, then addressing their sleep issues can set them on a path to getting healthy and achieving their victory.

Another study, by Dr. Michael Fitzpatrick, illustrated that patients with blocked nasal passages will have a

25 William Maixner et al., "Orofacial Pain Prospective Evaluation and Risk Assessment—the OPPERA Study," *J Pain* 12, no. 11 (November 2012); AE Sanders et al., "Sleep apnea symptoms and risk of temporomandibular disorder: OPPERA cohort," *J Dent Res* 92, no. 7 (May 2013).

26 Olmos, Steven, et al., "Headache and jaw locking comorbidity with daytime sleepiness," *American Journal of Dentistry*, vol. 29, no. 3 (June 2016): 161-165.

worsening of their OSA symptoms.[27] While it cannot absolutely be stated that a blocked nose will cause sleep apnea, we know that patients with blocked nasal passages will have worsening breathing while asleep. This illustrates the importance of doing a comprehensive exam and evaluating the entire respiratory pathway, from the tip of the nose all the way down to the epiglottis.

DONNA'S VICTORY

At Donna's first follow-up visit, two weeks after receiving her oral appliance, she stated that her pain level above the shoulders decreased from a nine to a three. Her tooth pain was gone, and her facial pain seemed to be gone, but she told us she was hesitant to admit that because she didn't think it was possible. After so many years of facial pain, she found it hard to believe that her problems might actually be resolving so quickly.

She also reported that she was no longer taking Benadryl to fall asleep, and that she didn't wake up repeatedly during the night anymore, but instead was waking at 5 a.m., rested and ready to start her day.

In two weeks' time, we were able to reduce facial pain that she'd had for forty years to a point where she was nearly ready to admit that it was nonexistent. Of course, we weren't done yet, but to see so much progress in such a short time was

---

27 Fitzpatrick, Michael, et al., "Effect of nasal or oral breathing route on upper airway resistance during sleep," *European Respiratory Journal*, no. 22 (2003): 827-832.

an encouraging indication of how treatment would go. And it was an added pleasure to have the patient on board, joining us in the confidence that the treatments would resolve her symptoms.

This chapter illustrates that the primary focus really should always be around identifying the origin of the patient's problem. In Donna's case, it was the airway issues and improving her breathing, which dramatically improved her quality of life. Often, breathing is not taken into consideration when the patient is getting evaluated by doctors, and this is something that is paramount in our treatment process with patients. Since everything in the body is interconnected, modern practitioners need to look not only deeper within their own areas of practice, but at the interrelationships between their specialty and other areas of medicine. Had we only focused on Donna's self-reported TMD, we likely would have had the same results that her previous providers and the forty years of treatment had yielded. It was only upon taking a step back and looking at the bigger picture of her situation that we were able to identify that the root cause of her problems was associated with her nighttime breathing—and the results speak for themselves. It seems almost too simple, but that is what is so rewarding about what I do.

Like Donna, many patients benefit from being treated with a team approach, which is why a sleep physician, ENT physician, nurse practitioner, chiropractor, and osteopathic physician are all part of our treatment team.

In Chapter 8, I will discuss some of the comprehensive therapy and treatment modalities that we use in our office and illustrate what many patients receive as part of the treatment plan with our team. Moving forward, let's look at a condition that causes some patients debilitating pain.

CHAPTER 7
TRIGEMINAL NEURALGIA:
DO WE ALWAYS NEED
MEDICATIONS OR SURGERIES?

Trigeminal neuralgia is a chronic pain condition that affects the trigeminal nerve, which is one of twelve cranial nerves that carry sensory and motor information from the face to the brain.

The trigeminal nerve has three branches, and classical trigeminal neuralgia is noted as severe stabbing neuropathic facial pain of the second and third divisions of the nerve. Together, those two branches, or divisions, stimulate the cheek, maxilla and mandible, top and bottom lip, teeth and gums, and side of the nose.[28]

For people with trigeminal neuralgia, a mild stimulation to the face, such as from brushing their teeth, applying makeup, or even the wind blowing, may trigger a jolt of excruciating pain.[29] At first, patients usually experience short, mild attacks, but these can progress into longer, more frequent bouts of stabbing pain.

Trigeminal neuralgia affects women more than men, and it is more likely to occur in people who are over age fifty. It's estimated that some fifteen thousand people suffer from it but from experience treating this for years, I suspect that number is grossly underestimated.[30]

Betty was one of those afflicted with trigeminal neuralgia. She was seventy years old when she first came in for a consultation. Her chief complaints included symptoms of trigeminal neuralgia along with facial pain, pain when chewing, limited ability to open her mouth, and jaw joint noises.

For Betty, her victory was clear: to find a cause for the pain. She wanted to get rid of the pain because it kept her from being able to babysit her grandkids or even spend a

---

28 "Trigeminal Neuralgia Fact Sheet," National Institute of Neurological Disorders and Stroke, accessed February 20, 2018, https://www.ninds.nih.gov/Disorders/Patient-Caregiver-Education/Fact-Sheets/Trigeminal-Neuralgia-Fact-Sheet.

29 "Trigeminal neuralgia," May Clinic, accessed February 20, 2018, https://www.mayoclinic.org/diseases-conditions/trigeminal-neuralgia/symptoms-causes/syc-20353344.

30 "Trigeminal Neuralgia," Johns Hopkins Health Library, accessed February 20, 2018, https://www.hopkinsmedicine.org/healthlibrary/conditions/nervous_system_disorders/trigeminal_neuralgia_134,66.

little time playing with them. She could not take care of them alone, and that was killing her.

Betty's first visit was in September 2017. At that time, she had pain on the left side of her face, starting at her ear and extending all the way across her cheek to

——— **VICTORY** ———

For Betty, her victory was clear: to find a cause for the pain.

the midline. She described the pain as an electrical shock—a sharp, stabbing, debilitating pain. Since her pain was nine on a scale of ten, she said it kept her from feeling alive. She told us she prayed for help and relief, and that's when her physical therapist at a hospital over sixty miles away recommended that she come see me for evaluation. As you will read in a bit, sixty miles was not a big deal for her to travel to see us.

Before being diagnosed with trigeminal neuralgia, Betty had undergone root canals in two teeth—one upper, one lower—on the left side of her face, thinking they were the cause of the pain. She even had one of those teeth extracted, but that still didn't provide any relief. Then, in the spring of 2017, she was formally diagnosed with trigeminal neuralgia at the Mayo Clinic in Rochester, Minnesota. They completed a thorough workup on Betty that included CT scans, an MRI, and a clinical evaluation. It was recommended that she undergo microvascular decompression surgery to address her trigeminal neuralgia.

In May 2017, four months before becoming a patient of mine, Betty underwent the surgery with a titanium mesh cranioplasty. The surgery involved drilling into the occipital bone at the base of the skull and entering the space of the cranial vault, that space inside the skull that houses the brain. Betty's trigeminal nerve was being compressed by the superior and anterior cerebral artery, and the surgeons placed Teflon felt in between the artery and the nerve to reduce compression on the nerve. The surgery went without complication, and titanium mesh was placed with bone wax through the access point of the skull.

The goal of the procedure was to relieve the compression of the trigeminal nerve centrally, within the cranial vault, and eliminate the trigeminal pain in the periphery, or the areas of her face where she was experiencing pain. The procedure involved relocating the blood vessels that were in contact with the nerve root under her brain to prevent the nerve from malfunctioning. If the vein is compressing the nerve, the surgeon may remove it. Part of the trigeminal nerve may also be cut during this procedure in hopes to relive the pain if once inside, it is noted that the arteries aren't actually pressing on the nerve.

Microvascular decompression can eliminate or reduce pain, but sometimes the pain reoccurs within four years. This is what Betty was told before the surgery. Following Betty's surgery, she reported profound relief for two weeks. Then the pain returned just as before. She returned to the Mayo Clinic, and a second procedure was recommended and completed in August. This second procedure was gamma knife radiation, a.k.a. stereotactic radiosurgery, directed at the trigeminal nerve. The delivery of radiation to the trigeminal nerve is image guided and completed under sedation. The surgical report I reviewed stated that the procedure went well, without complication.

A month later, Betty was in our office for the first time looking for answers because her pain abruptly returned despite the two surgeries completed by very talented and well-intended surgeons from the esteemed Mayo Clinic.

THE CONNECTION TO SBD

I decided to include this chapter because we routinely see patients presenting with trigeminal neuralgia or with symptoms indicating that it may be present. Every case I have personally seen and treated in my office has met these two criteria: patients are in the fifth decade of life, and they are suffering from sleep breathing disorder (SBD). Often they don't know they have SBD, so we have to order appropriate testing, but in my practice, we have always found that to be present in these cases. As Dr. Olmos eloquently explains in his paper "Chasing Pain: Diagnosing and Treating Trigeminal Neuralgia in General Dentistry," if the problem is a peripheral entrapment, we must treat the nerve in the periphery. That's where intraoral orthotics and photobiomodulation therapy (PBMT) are potential solutions, versus medications and surgeries.[31]

---

31 Steven Olmos, "Chasing Pain: Diagnosing and Treating Trigeminal Neuralgia in General Dentistry," *DentalTown, January 2016*, http://

In Betty's case, two quite invasive surgeries, one which involved boring a hole through the base of the skull behind the ear, proved to be ineffective, since the problem wasn't residing in the cranial vault or in the base of the skull. Instead, it was residing as an entrapment of the nerve as it coursed through the muscles of the face.

In considering the connection between trigeminal neuralgia and SBDs, it's also important to note that 26 percent of the American population is reportedly at high risk for SBD.[32] The case study with Betty illustrates these incident relationships between SBDs and trigeminal neuralgia, so we encourage those suffering with facial pain not only to get an accurate diagnosis, but to have a treatment plan that's tailored to addressing where the pain is coming from. Now I'm not saying there is no role for these surgeries, as specific cases may certainly require them, but in my patient population, I have not seen the need given the patients who have presented to me for treatment.

BETTY'S VICTORY

During that first visit with Betty, we completed our comprehensive exam and imaging. Our exam revealed quite substantial findings. Betty was suffering from osteoarthritis in both

www.dentaltown.com/Images/Dentaltown/magimages/0116/
PAINpg34.pdf

32 "Rising prevalence of sleep apnea in U.S. threatens public health,"
American Academy of Sleep Medicine, news release, September
29, 2014, accessed February 20, 2018, https://aasm.org/
rising-prevalence-of-sleep-apnea-in-u-s-threatens-public-health.

condyles of her mandible, she had a severe dental abscess on one of her back teeth, and she had a deviated nasal septum to the left, which impeded her ability to breathe through her nose. We immediately referred her to an ENT physician and an endodontist for further evaluation of these findings.

Our evaluation also revealed profound risk indicators for SBD. These included snoring, fatigue, tongue scalloping, bruxism, narrow airway, nasal blockage and congestion, and frequent awakening.

We wholeheartedly agreed with the diagnosis of trigeminal neuralgia. Donna's symptoms certainly fit the classical description without a doubt, but we also referred her for a diagnostic sleep study since we felt that her chronic sleep disturbance and bruxism were associated with her trigeminal neuralgia and impingement of the nerve.

Although with Betty we arrived at the same diagnosis as Mayo Clinic, our treatment plan was quite different. We elected to treat her in the face (the periphery), rather than with the centrally directed surgeries that proved not to be effective. We surmised that her bruxism, or constant clenching and grinding throughout the night, was so aggressive that it destroyed the bone in her TM joint. If it was aggressive enough to destroy the bone, it was completely plausible that the nerves were impinging her trigeminal nerve, producing the pain. After all, what did she have to lose—we weren't going to do another brain surgery.

Our treatment plan consisted of oral appliance therapy to decompress the TM joints and reduce her strong contraction forces at nighttime. The Mayo Clinic had treated the trigeminal nerve as it exited the brain, but the problem was an impingement in her face through the masseter muscle, where the nerve courses. We treated it at the source of the entrapment in the face rather than at the base of the skull. In this case, that proved to be effective almost immediately.

We also planned PBMT to help create an ideal environment for healing and repair of her damaged nerve. PBMT is also known as laser therapy, low-level therapy, or cold laser therapy. I'll share more details about PBMT in Chapter 8.

Betty's treatment began in mid-October with delivery of the sleep orthotic and PBMT directed at the trigeminal nerve. The sleep orthotic was designed to stabilize her TM joint to treat the arthritis there and to take pressure off the nerve entrapment. As we initiated treatment, we ordered a sleep study to investigate her suspected SBD.

At her first follow-up visit two weeks later, Betty reported that her pain was reduced from a nine to a four on a ten-point scale. Specifically, she reported a 75 percent reduction of her trigeminal neuralgia, facial pain, and pain when chewing. She also reported a 60 percent improvement of her limited range of motion when opening her mouth. Fast-forward to mid-November 2017, Betty reported her pain level to be a one out of ten, and all her symptoms were reduced by 90 percent.

Betty is now in treatment with a sleep physician for her SBD, and she continues to wear the orthotic we created for her every night. Thankfully, within a month, we were able to resolve her trigeminal neuralgia without the use of medications or surgery.

Best of all, Betty can now babysit her grandkids and get down on the floor with them and play. "I feel alive again," she told us at her last appointment—nothing beats that feeling for us as well.

As I complete this book in May 2018, Betty's pain has been completely resolved since November, with no flare-ups or recurrences. That assures us that we treated the source of the problem and that Betty will be able to continue playing with her grandkids—and living a wonderful life—free of debilitating facial pain.

CHAPTER 8
COMPREHENSIVE THERAPY AND TREATMENT MODALITIES

Is there a "magic bullet"? Yes, there is!

Nancy was referred to me by a physiatrist (a physical medicine and rehab physician) for problems with sleep and pain. The physiatrist was a seasoned doctor of forty-plus years who had been treating Nancy with acupuncture for her chronic pain for over two years. While they were having success with reducing her pain, the physician thought more could be done. He and I spoke extensively about the incidence of obstructive sleep apnea (OSA), how chronic pain disrupts sleep, and the relationship between insomnia and sleep apnea. He thought we could help, and he told me,

"I learned so much from you that I wasn't taught in medical school or my forty years of continuing education."

Now, this physician had to listen to me, because he's my father, Dr. Roger Klauer. Nonetheless, just as he has made me a better practitioner, it is humbling to know that I have also impacted his practice of medicine in a positive manner.

Nancy was having trouble falling asleep, and when she finally did, she'd constantly toss and turn and wake up repeatedly throughout the night. Mornings were always a challenge—she'd wake unrefreshed, and spent many days dealing with chronic sleepiness, headaches, and pain, the latter of which was finally diagnosed as fibromyalgia. At age fifty-five, Nancy had already been taking medication and treatment for chronic pain for about ten years and was also medicating her high blood pressure and gastroesophageal reflux (GERD).

Her victory? A good night's sleep. She didn't even consider pain relief among her victories. She just accepted it as part of life. It really pains me to know that some patients have become so desensitized when there are solutions available.

—— **VICTORY** ——

Nancy's victory? A good night's sleep. She didn't even consider pain relief among her victories. She just accepted it as part of life.

Rather quickly, our comprehensive examination pointed to undiagnosed sleep apnea as the culprit for her problems. Yes, her breathing at night was one of our highest concerns—no surprise there. Again, nothing trumps the importance of breathing—or sleep, for that matter. In addition to the symptoms, we found that Nancy was a heavy snorer, had a scalloped tongue, and had profound nasal obstructions that grossly inhibited her ability to breathe through her nose.

Still, Nancy was a little apprehensive about undergoing a sleep test: "I don't sleep, so what will a sleep test show?" she wanted to know. A sleep test, I explained, would show us what was happening when she did fall asleep.

It's a good thing she came in for consultation with us and then ultimately agreed to the sleep study. Her results showed that she was waking from sleep fifty-four times an hour due to a breathing event. Her AHI was fifty-four! Nearly every single minute of the little sleep she did get was disrupted by a waking episode. When she was able to get into REM sleep—that deep sleep that helps with memory consolidation and cognitive function—she was waking even more often, up to eighty times an hour. So in that most valuable stage of sleep, she was waking more than once every minute. No wonder she was tired and miserable in the morning. I wouldn't want to fall asleep if I knew that I would stop breathing more than once a minute—I would do everything I could to stay awake and not suffocate. And that's exactly what Nancy was doing each night.

Nancy was excited about the results of her sleep test. For the first time in years, something quantifiable was identified as the cause of her symptoms. Better yet, it was something that could be treated. That diagnosis of severe OSA by a sleep physician helped us develop a clear treatment plan for Nancy.

Nancy's situation was so severe that it took several modalities to treat her, including a referral to a sleep physician who was also an ENT (Dr. Doug Liepert, who wrote the foreword to this book).

As I've mentioned, sometimes a few practitioners must work closely together and constantly keep the channels of communication open so that the patient can achieve optimal health. Other providers that we often work with include ENTs, neurologists, sleep physicians, osteopathic physicians, chiropractors, family practice physicians, nurses, and physical therapists.

After so many years of suffering and pain, Nancy was happy to comply with our referral recommendations.

THE MAGIC BULLET

Often when people present with chronic pain and sleep problems, we're asked, "Is there a magic bullet?" There is a magic bullet, and it is attainable for most of our patients. Here's what it took to get Nancy to the finish line. Keep in mind that Nancy was dealing with fifty-plus years of suffering, suffocating, and long-term destruction. It took her a long time to get unhealthy and so broken down, so it would take several modalities to get her health back.

Orthotics

With TMD, the treatment modality we often employ is the use of an orthotic. In the TMD world, orthotics, splints, mouth guards, and appliances are often used interchangeably, but an orthotic is very different from a mouth guard or a splint. A mouth guard or splint is a static device that is used as a shim between the teeth and/or just something to grind on and protect the teeth. Splints and mouth guards aren't intended to be used while eating. An orthotic is intended to be used during eating, chewing, and speaking, and to be worn throughout the day to protect the TM joints from harm by keeping them in an orthopedically stable position.

An FDA-approved sleep appliance for OSA is often referred to as a "mandibular repositioning appliance" (MRA), "mandibular advancement device" (MAD), "oral appliance therapy" (OAT), or a "sleep appliance." These appliances are designed to prevent retrusion of the mandible to prevent it and the soft palate and the tongue from collapsing into the airway during sleep. However, if a patient has existing TMD symptoms and OSA, we can often make an FDA-approved sleep appliance that treats both sets of symptoms. People with OSA have a 3.6 times greater likelihood of having TMD.[33]

For maximum benefit when using these modalities, the sinuses and nasal passages must be healthy and clear. If the nose is blocked, the facial muscles will tighten up and

---

33 Steven Olmos, "Comorbidities of Chronic Facial Pain and Obstructive Sleep Apnea," *Current Opinion in Pulmonary Medicine* 22, no. 6 (November 2016): 570-5.

cause excess strain and an open-mouth posture. That strains the mastication muscles, those muscles used for chewing. If pushing on the muscles that move the jaw causes noticeable discomfort, and that is normal, that means there is chronic congestion present causing muscles to be tight and sore, and to activate/fire too frequently.

CPAP

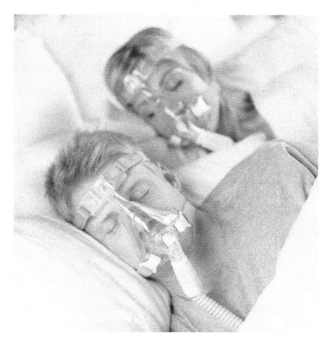

A continuous positive airway pressure machine (CPAP) is a device that blows air through the nose and down the throat to help keep the airway open during sleep. The OSA sufferer wears a mask on their face at night that is connected by a hose to the CPAP. The American Academy of Sleep Medicine (AASM) recommends CPAPs for patients with severe sleep apnea. For patients with mild to moderate sleep apnea, the AASM recommends oral appliances or CPAPs, based on patient preference or clinical evaluation.

Since Nancy's sleep apnea was so severe, the clinical guidelines recommended a CPAP as the first line of treatment. While many patients benefit from a CPAP, many also struggle with compliance, or regular use of the machine. In fact, research has found compliance with a CPAP to be as low as 17 percent.[34] On the flip side, compliance with oral appliances is typically 90 percent or better.[35] I don't want to give a negative impression of CPAP therapy, since it benefits many patients, but it's nice to know that there are several options for treating people suffering from these debilitating disorders.

Combination Therapy

Often with a CPAP, the patient's mandible still retracts back into their throat when they sleep, so their CPAP pressure must be extremely high. Using an appliance to stabilize the mandible allows for lower CPAP pressure and tends to increase compliance. Nancy needed combination therapy because her case was so severe and she initially struggled with the CPAP.

---

34 Weaver, Terri and Ronald Grunstein, "Adherence to Continuous Positive Airway Pressure Therapy," Proceedings of the American Thoracic Society, vol. 5 (2008): 173-178.

35 Ibid.

Surgical Techniques

There are surgical techniques that can help patients with more severe cases of TMD and/or OSA.

According to the American Academy of Sleep Medicine (AASM) Clinical Practice Parameters and Guidelines, oral appliances and CPAPs should be attempted first, prior to any surgical procedures, so we usually exhaust all conservative modalities prior to moving in that direction.[36] When surgery is necessary, we have a network of very talented oral surgeons that we turn to.

Since the success rate with TM joint surgeries is extremely low, we rarely recommend these; they are reserved as secondary or tertiary options for patients. Just as with CPAP, I don't want to give a negative impression of surgery of the TM joints, but in my practice, we rarely need to turn to surgery to achieve our patients' victories for the TMD. Now, with developmental abnormalities or trauma, then surgical procedures are sometimes needed and recommended.

Surgical procedures for OSA are on occasion used in conjunction with our treatment. These surgeries include removal of the tonsils and adenoids, partial dissection of the tongue, and maxillomandibular advancement, which involves moving the maxilla and mandible forward to help open the airway. Maxillomandibular advancement has as

---

36 Clete A. Kushida et al., "Practice Parameters for the Treatment of Snoring and Obstructive Sleep Apnea with Oral Appliances: An Update for 2005," *SLEEP* 29, no. 2 (2006): 240-3.

much as a 99 percent success rate but is extremely costly and takes some time to recover, so it is reserved as a last resort.[37]

There are also older surgical techniques involving removal of part of the soft palate and uvula. However, since these are successful less than 20 percent of the time, they are rarely used anymore.

Trigger Points

Many people are familiar with the term "trigger points." A trigger point is an area in the connective tissue (fascia) or muscle that is painful when compressed. This compression can cause referred pain to other areas of the body. Drs. Janet Travell and David Simons define trigger point in their "bible" on the subject, *Myofascial Pain and Dysfunction: The Trigger Point Manual, Second Edition, Volume 1*, as: "A primary myofascial trigger point is a central myofascial trigger point that was … activated directly by acute or chronic overload or repetitive overuse of the muscle in which it occurs and was not activated because of trigger point activity in another muscle."

---

37 Paolo Ronchi, "Maxillomandibular Advancement in Obstructive Sleep Apnea Syndrome Patients: a Retrospective Study on the Sagittal Cephalometric Variables," *Journal of Oral & Maxillofacial Research* 4, no. 2 (April-June 2013): e5, accessed on U.S. Library of Medicine National Institutes of Health, February 20, 2018, https://www.ncbi.nlm.nih.gov/pmc/articles/PMC3886110/.

TRIGGER POINTS

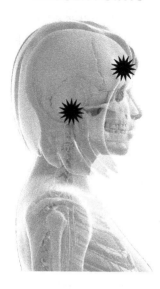

In other words, a trigger point results from overuse of the muscle. A knot forms within the muscle and can refer pain to other sites of that muscle or associated muscles. Yes, pain in one area of the muscle can refer pain to a completely different area.

It's very important to be able to identify trigger points in patients, because TM joint problems, breathing problems, chronic forward head posture, car accidents, and different injuries can cause the development of trigger points. Until those trigger points are released, patients will experience pain or discomfort. What is just as important as identifying the trigger point is identifying the origin of it—what overuse is occurring to produce the trigger point.

According to Drs. Travell and Simons: "One well-performed trigger point injection can fully inactivate a trigger

point immediately." However, the authors say, identifying and releasing trigger points is not for everyone—patients with fibromyalgia and trigger points sometimes do not have the profound results of patients with just trigger points.

We commonly treat trigger points in the head and neck, since those directly relate to the symptoms we see. Therapies that we use to treat trigger points include injections of an anesthetic solution to help dissipate the trigger point and restore proper function to the muscle or muscle groups being treated. The trigger point technique is extremely valuable because it's very effective and conservative. The injection is superficial, staying clear of joint spaces or anatomical danger zones that can harm a patient. And the injection itself is not a caustic substance, it is simply an anesthetic solution. Other forms of trigger point therapy that we use include manual pressure and laser therapy.

Laser Therapy

Laser therapy, commonly known as cold laser therapy, low level laser therapy, or photobiomodulation therapy (PBMT), uses light to enhance the body's natural healing processes. Lasers have been used in medicine for many years. PBMT is not a surgical laser, but rather a therapeutic, non-cutting laser that does not cause pain when applied. Yes, surprisingly, shining a light on body structures decreases pain and increases healing.

The light used in this therapy is applied to the skin, allowing the light energy (photons) to penetrate tissue where it interacts with various molecules (chromophores), resulting in different biological effects.

PBMT has photochemical, photothermal, and photo-mechanical interactions with the body that produce healing results. The photochemical interaction is direct transfer of energy to the biological substrates (chromophores). The photothermal interaction is conversion of light energy into heat, which promotes healing. And the photomechanical interaction is the absorption of light involving the formation of mechanical waves. This light energy can be directed over specific parts of the body to produce therapeutic results that are essential in the healing process.

To get it to the cellular level, the laser increases production of:

- ribonucleic acid (RNA), a molecule in the body that helps the body use proteins;

- ATP synthesis, which helps cells function better;

- macrophage activity, helping to repair tissues;

- cell proliferation, or the growing of healthy cells; and

- extracellular matrix production by fibroblasts and chondrocytes, which helps in healing.

PBMT also releases growth factors (for cell regulation), causes proliferation of T and B lymphocytes (types of immune system cells), and decreases mass effects in bone marrow. Those are some very technical explanations of laser activity, but they illustrate that there's a lot going on at the physiological level as the laser is being applied to a patient's skin. PBMT is extremely safe and effective, and we have great references and resources for patients looking to learn and understand more about the treatment.

Basically, the laser has three main therapeutic effects: it decreases pain, speeds up the healing process, and helps repair broken nerves. In treating inflammatory conditions, PBMT is essential in attaining the results and healing for our patients. PBMT laser treatments range from three to fifteen minutes, and the application is comfortable without excessive heat or discomfort to the patient. I honestly could not practice without it. Our office currently has three units that are used all day.

Prolotherapy

Dr. George S. Hackett is considered to be the father of prolotherapy. He began using this technique around 1939, and it is currently used by many physicians and dentists like myself. Prolotherapy dates as far back as the gladiator days, when hot metal tips were inserted into joint capsules to repair strained and sprained ligaments—thankfully, that's not how the treatment works today.

Prolotherapy is the name some people use for a type of medical intervention for musculoskeletal pain that causes proliferation of collagen fibers, such as those found in ligaments and tendons, as well as shortening of those fibers. Collagen is composed of connective tissues that support the body's structures. The "prolo" in prolotherapy comes from "proliferative."

Other therapists have referred to this type of treatment as "sclerotherapy." "Sclera" comes from the Greek word *sklero*, which means "harden." Sclerotherapy refers to the same type of medical interventions as prolotherapy—interventions that produce a proliferation of collagen fibers and thus a hardening of the tissue treated.

Prolotherapy is a valuable technique for helping with stretched, strained, and sprained ligaments around the jaw joint capsule and associated attachments to the mandible. These ligaments often get stretched from chronic, repetitive injuries (micro trauma) or from accidents (macro trauma). Selective injection into the areas where the ligaments connect to bone produce hardening or scar tissue to form and repair the stretched ligaments. Prolotherapy provides considerable relief and helps with healing following an injury.

Prolotherapy is not used on all patients, but it's a great technique to finalize the healing process. Prolotherapy is widely used by musculoskeletal pain physicians in other parts of the body to repair chronically strained ligaments and tendons. I am fortunate to work closely with the author of the best-known medical textbook on prolotherapy, Dr. Mark Cantieri. His book, *Principles of Prolotherapy*, is a great resource for physicians and dentists learning these techniques. I have trained with him one-on-one and we co-treat patients daily.

Myofunctional Therapy

As William Proffit's textbook *Contemporary Orthodontics* states, "Respiratory needs are the primary determinant of the posture of the jaws, tongue, and head. Therefore, it seems entirely reasonable that an altered respiratory pattern, such as breathing through the mouth rather than the nose, could change the posture of the head, jaw, teeth, and tongue."

Myofunctional therapy is the study and treatment of oral and facial muscles as they relate to speech, dentition, chewing, collection, swallowing, and overall mental and physical health. Proper tongue function is necessary for optimal nasal breathing. The tongue can be trained to rest in the proper position in the mouth to facilitate adequate nasal breathing rather than mouth breathing. Treatment usually includes a series of activities aimed at training and retraining the muscles of the face and oral cavity. These can't be learned overnight, but rather with time.

Activities for this can be supplemented temporarily with oral appliances that are designed to help patients develop the proper dental arch and adequate position of the tongue. Active treatment typically encompasses anywhere from three months to six months, followed by maintenance visits and a form of learning known as habituation. We have two trained and certified myofunctional therapists in our office who provide this service for our patients who need retraining of the oral, facial, and tongue muscles.

Nutrition

As we treat patients with chronic pain, we often have to draw attention to their food intake, because it can play a major role in their disease process. Patients often consume foods that work against their body's ability to heal or, in fact, create problems for our patients.

Generally speaking, we recommend a low-inflammatory diet. Excessive inflammation is the precursor to all disease processes, so anything we can do to lower inflammation can help the patient. While there are several good "diets," and a lot depends on the specific patient, a low-inflammatory diet means eating a diet of primarily unprocessed foods that is low in added sugar and artificial, manufactured substances. A clean diet with a good balance of protein and vegetables is what we strive for with most of our patients. Adequate water consumption and avoidance of artificial food additives and chemicals typically allows people to accelerate through the healing process.

These days, it is hard to know what we are eating, so we spend a great deal of time educating patients on their dietary choices. For patients with extreme circumstances, we have wonderful wellness partners in the community that we can turn to. Ultimately, we encourage our patients to read labels and understand what they are eating and how food can make or break their health.

The value of nutrition in treating a patient with chronic pain and sleep problems cannot be overstated. Often, the problems people are dealing with are reactions and sensitivities to the foods they are eating, and they don't even know it. By eliminating those foods, patients can begin to see results.

Wellness Coaching

While eating healthy is crucial to healing, it's also important to be physically and mentally fit. We offer wellness coaching through specially trained practitioners who help guide patients in adapting a healthy lifestyle, encouraging them to achieve and master the Triad of Health.

With all of the aforementioned therapeutic modalities, it's important that the evaluations and treatments are rendered by practitioners who have treated numerous patients and are keeping up with what's going on in the field. It's up to the practitioner to be responsible for using only methods that have been validated as effective by research studies.

NANCY'S VICTORY

In Nancy's situation, getting a diagnosis of sleep apnea was key to treatment. That's why we always evaluate a patient's breathing during their first visit. Since sleep comprises one-third of each day, discovering Nancy's problem was essential to achieving her victory.

Considering the severity of her OSA, CPAP was the first treatment initiated. However, it proved to be ineffective, because Nancy could not tolerate wearing the machine throughout the night. At the recommendation of her sleep physician, she returned to our office to initiate oral appliance therapy, and we designed a custom oral appliance for her to use while sleeping to treat her OSA.

Once Nancy got comfortable with her oral appliance, she reattempted CPAP therapy at a lower pressure—using both treatments is known as combination therapy, discussed earlier in this chapter. The oral appliance allowed us to reduce her CPAP pressure, making it easier to tolerate the treatment. After the first night, Nancy noted a profound improvement in her ability to tolerate the CPAP mask every night. That's what we call a success!

We also recommended that she visit an ENT physician to repair the obstruction in her nasal airway. Once that correction was made, her ability to breathe improved greatly both day and night.

Lastly, but arguably just as important, we set her up with a wellness coach, who went over diet guidelines and exercises with her to help her be physically and mentally fit.

Through our coordinated care involving a sleep physician, ENT, wellness coach, and our oral appliance therapy, Nancy was able to achieve her victory.

Admittedly, her results took a little time; they did not happen overnight. Nancy's case was more on the severe end, but it illustrates so many facets of what we can achieve. Within a year of starting treatment, Nancy went from being extremely tired, never sleeping through the night, and consistently waking without feeling refreshed to having a far greater quality of life—she had more energy, got more sleep, and woke up feeling refreshed. She was also on a healthy diet, which helped her lose and keep off *sixty pounds*, and she'd reduced the number of pain meds she was taking. Her severe sleep apnea was adequately treated via a CPAP and an oral appliance, both of which she wears every night and says she cannot sleep without.

I continue to see Nancy on an annual basis to ensure that she is maintaining her victory and enjoying life. Three years posttreatment, she continues to feel great. She has even become a spokesperson for our office and routinely attends our wellness events and workshops to help motivate patients who are having the same struggles as she had. She proudly shares her story and we are just as proud of her.

Nancy's case demonstrates how sleep apnea can produce years of pain and suffering. Her inability to breathe properly at nighttime and get adequate sleep was ruining her life. I estimate that she had been suffering from sleep apnea for at least thirty years.

That doesn't have to be the case for other people. Intervention and prevention at an earlier age can identify breathing and structural problems in youth, helping to stave off years of pain and suffering, medical expenses, and complications of issues. In the next chapter, I will discuss how TMD and OSA problems of adulthood can often be avoided if the structural issues of the mouth are addressed in childhood.

CHAPTER 9
TODAY CAN MAKE ALL THE DIFFERENCE TOMORROW

If we can treat children early enough, we can potentially prevent problems later in life.

At age five, Sean had his tonsils and adenoids removed to relieve his snoring, asthma, allergies, and frequent illnesses. Initially, that helped a bit, but his symptoms returned over a two-year span, and his mother brought him in to see us. She had become extremely concerned because Sean would stop breathing during sleep, but the surgeon who had removed his tonsils had no further recommendations for treatment. At five years old, Sean was taking many different medications—for his allergies and ADHD, and some to be able to sleep at night.

Sean's victory was to sleep through the night and determine whether his ADHD was related to his poor sleep.

—— **VICTORY** ——

Sean's victory was to sleep through the night and determine whether his ADHD was related to his poor sleep.

Inflamed tonsil and adenoid tissue, unfortunately, is somewhat common in children. Now, just because it is common does not make it normal—keep that in mind. That lymphatic tissue is essential for immunity and is required in pediatric patients as they grow and develop, but if it becomes too hypertrophic (enlarged) and inflamed, it can obstruct the airway and require removal. In fact, removal is a common recommendation without ever understanding what caused the tissue to become inflamed in the first place. There is a reason the tissue becomes inflamed, and it is our job as practitioners to find it. In Sean's case, it was his perpetual mouth breathing, which we noted during his clinical exam.

A comprehensive evaluation of Sean determined that he needed to undergo a diagnostic sleep study. Currently, the American Academy of Pediatrics' Practice Parameters and Clinical Guidelines recommends that all children be screened for snoring during medical visits, and that any child with snoring undergo a diagnostic sleep study. Furthermore, the American Academy of Sleep Medicine recommends that children complete their sleep study under direct supervision at a sleep center. While home sleep studies are FDA approved for children, it can be hard for them to complete the test successfully without supervision.

We ordered the study for Sean, and the results were astounding. Despite his tonsils and adenoids being removed, he was still suffering from obstructive sleep apnea (OSA). The study showed that he had three episodes an hour and that his breathing would slow to the point of stopping, at which point he would wake up from sleep. Furthermore, during REM, or deep sleep, he was awakened nine times an hour. Again, REM is crucial for cognitive function development, which is extremely important in growing children.

We presented Sean's treatment options to his mom. Since he had already undergone the first line of treatment—having his tonsils and adenoids removed—another option was a CPAP. While CPAP machines are great tools and necessary for children at times, prescribing it would likely condemn him to using it for the rest of his life. Plus, the retractive forces of the CPAP would hinder his facial development—since the mask would attach to his head and pull backward on the face, it would prevent his face from growing and developing forward as nature intended. We try our best to avoid retractive forces on the facial structures of pediatric patients.

The other option for Sean was orthopedic expansion of the maxilla and mandible. By developing his maxilla—which, again, is the bottom of the nose—Sean would be able to breathe better and have greater nasal volume. In fact, the amount of increased width achieved in the nose would increase the flow of air to the fourth power. By increasing the width of his mandible, there would be more room for his tongue, helping it to rest upward and forward in the palate and prevent it from crowding his airway. These measures to develop his jaw laterally and forward would allow his airway to develop to its full genetic potential. As humans, we have a genotype and a phenotype. Our genotype is our DNA, our biological identity. Our phenotype is the physical expression of our genotype based on the environmental factors we are exposed to. We can alter our phenotype based upon the interactions of our genes and our environment.

The results of the sleep study were good news, because we had an answer to Sean's problems. With his mom's approval, we were able to initiate treatment and begin fabricating his upper and lower expanders right away. We also had the encouragement from the sleep physician to initiate expansion rather than go the CPAP route. We were excited about his treatment because we knew we were going to start transforming his life right then. His treatment today will make all the difference tomorrow.

SLEEP IS ESSENTIAL TO GROWTH AND DEVELOPMENT

Medical literature shows that 10 percent of children are diagnosed with ADHD,[38] and that 10 percent are diagnosed

---

38 "Attention-Deficit / Hyperactivity Disorder (ADHD)," Centers for Disease Control and Prevention, accessed February 20, 2018, https://www.cdc.gov/ncbddd/adhd/data.html.

with OSA or sleep breathing disorder (SBD).[39] Is it a coincidence that these rates are identical? I do not propose that ADHD does not exist, not by any means, but I do propose that a great deal can go wrong in an individual whose breathing is altered while they are growing and developing. After all, sleep is a crucial time for growth and development. Dr. Darius Loghmanee, a pediatric sleep physician and medical director of six Chicagoland Pediatric Sleep Centers with Advocate Health Care, is a good friend of mine. In a recent lecture to our local community, he advocated for better sleep health. He eloquently explained that the top three symptoms of ADHD are:

- Inattention

- Hyperactivity

- Poor temper

He then went on to describe the top three symptoms of sleepiness in children:

- Inattention

- Hyperactivity

- Poor temper

Again, I'm not proposing that all ADHD symptoms are sleep problems. I am proposing that we better ensure there is

---

39 James Chan, Jennifer Edman, and Peter Koltai, "Obstructive Sleep Apnea in Children," *American Family Physician* 69, no. 5 (March 1, 2004): 1147–1155, https://www.aafp.org/afp/2004/0301/p1147.html

adequate sleep being achieved before initiating pharmaceutical treatment for children with symptoms of ADHD.

Take Sean, for example. In his most crucial stage of sleep, he was waking up nine times an hour. Ask any mother if you can conduct an experiment that involves waking up her child nine times an hour—and feel free to share her response with me. I asked my wife that question and she laughed at me, then issued a few threats—the experiment went no further.

Drs. Kevin L. Boyd and Stephen H. Sheldon wrote a great chapter in a medical textbook explaining the incidence of pediatric sleep-disordered breathing (another term for SBD) and its relationship to facial development. Here are some excerpts from their work:

> *Pediatric sleep-disordered breathing (SDB) is a pathological condition associated with a wide range of clinical symptoms, historical evidence, dentofacial physical examination findings, environmental components and genetic and/or epigenetic factors. Recently published controlled studies indicate a close association between pediatric SDB/OSA and neurocognitive impairments such as ADD/ADHD and other behavioral disorders. Many of the various physical characteristics associated with a high prevalence of pediatric SDB/OSA are also strongly associated with a number of pediatric dentofacial abnormalities; the relationship between pediatric SDB/OSA and*

the developing jaws and facial structures is also well described. [40]

Drs. Boyd and Sheldon write that physical features and facial developments can be risk indicators for development of SBD and cognitive dysfunctions in children as they grow and develop.

There are a number of factors that are known about facial development. For starters, dentofacial malocclusion is a risk indicator for OSA—if a patient has a narrow dental arch, crooked teeth, or open-mouth posture, they're at risk for developing OSA.

Also, since the agricultural revolution, craniofacial volume has steadily decreased. With the introduction of industrialized farming, facial and airway volumes have consistently decreased—faces have become smaller and nasal passages have become narrower. That is likely due to the lesser physical challenges posed to the developing palatal suture complex during infancy and early childhood. The palatal suture complex refers to the seams in the cranial bones that run along the roof of the mouth. Addressing development issues with these cranial sutures during childhood can, again, make all the difference tomorrow.

According to Boyd and Sheldon:

With ever accumulating physical evidence from anthropological studies, combined with advances in

---

40　Kevin L. Boyd and Stephen H. Sheldon, "Childhood Sleep-Disorder Breathing: A Dental Perspective," in *Principles and Practice of Pediatric Sleep Medicine*, Sheldon et al. (Elsevier Saunders: 2014): 273.

the newly emerging scientific disciplines of epigenetics and evolutionary medicine, it can be stated with a reasonable degree of scientific certainty that malocclusion is not primarily a genetically determined disease entity. Rather, malocclusion is better described as a WD (Western disease) *that is primarily mediated through a gene-environment interaction that follows a fairly predictable pattern of pathological progression: initially, most WDs are preventable so long as genetically predisposed individuals are identified before early phenotypic expression of the disease is obvious.*[41]

So, Drs. Boyd and Sheldon point to environment, more so than genetics, as being the cause of malformation of the maxilla and mandible, mouth, and teeth. With each generation of narrower faces and maxilla and mandible, the genotype is affected. Again, genotype is DNA, a person's biological identity. Those changes can even affect future generations—that is the study of epigenetics, a phenomenon that really takes an entire book to discuss. The point being: If we identify these problems in children early enough, we can change the disease progression and alter their growth and development, breathing, cognitive function, and ability to thrive. We can minimize the chances that malocclusion and

41   Kevin L. Boyd and Stephen H. Sheldon, "Childhood Sleep-Disorder Breathing: A Dental Perspective," in *Principles and Practice of Pediatric Sleep Medicine*, Sheldon et al. (Elsevier Saunders: 2014): 273.

limited facial growth will contribute to a child's poor sleep and breathing.

If a child grows to develop SBD and poor facial structure, their risk for TMD problems in the future also increases.

IDENTIFYING TMD AND OSA

In my practice, I often see adults who bring their children with them to appointments. Over the years, I began to see how those children would grow and develop if no intervention was done. So, I started treating kids basically out of necessity—I was treating parents whose children were beginning to suffer the same problems as the parents had in childhood, and those parents wanted the problems intervened at an earlier age.

Let's look as some of the common symptoms we see in pediatric patients dealing with TMD and/or sleep apnea. These include:

TMD AND/OR SLEEP APNEA SYMPTOMS IN CHILDREN

- headaches and migraines
- jaw and face pain
- bedwetting
- mouth breathing
- recurring ear infections
- impaired intelligence

- decreased performance/learning problems in school
- hyperactivity
- aggressiveness
- social isolation, withdrawal
- night terrors
- night sweats
- mood changes
- poor concentration

Headaches and migraines. Children diagnosed with migraines are 8.25 times more likely to have SBD. Whereas children diagnosed with chronic, tension-type headaches are 15.23 times more likely to have SBD.[42] If a child presents with headaches, facial pain, and ADHD-like symptoms, it's crucial to have a proper sleep evaluation and determine whether a diagnostic sleep study is an appropriate next step.

TMD pain and jaw joint noises. Dr. Olmos reported that one in six children and adolescents has clinical signs of TMD. Over 23 percent of preschool age children have pain when chewing and TM joint noises, and all that TM joint noise is pathologic. And in the United States and around the world, the prevalence of OSA is increasing. A total of 26 percent

---

42   Steven Olmos, "Pediatric severe apnea/obesity/TMD/headache —
      Class III," *Orthodontic Practice*, case study, vol. 7, no. 3.

of the American population is at high risk for OSA, and 57 percent of those are at high risk for OSA.[43] Thus, the earlier we can screen and treat these problems, the better chance we have of preventing them in adults.

Bed-wetting (nocturnal enuresis) is a hallmark indicator of OSA in children, because sleep problems can disrupt the hormones that regulate the urge to urinate. Once a child is past the age of potty training, ongoing bed-wetting needs to be addressed with a formal sleep evaluation to determine whether OSA is present.

Mouth breathing is another key indicator. It is normal to breathe through the nose, not through the mouth. Mouth breathing in children leads to a cascade of negative events, including less oxygen to the lungs, altered facial development, and episodes of hyperventilation (over-breathing) throughout the day. These cascades of events originating from mouth breathing causes us to get approximately 20 percent less oxygen to our tissue.

Pediatric patients with chronic mouth breathing also tend to have more upper respiratory congestion, and one of the common signs and symptoms of upper respiratory congestion is recurrent ear infections and buildup of inflammation inside the ear. Because they're mouth breathing

---

43   Steven Olmos, "Comorbidities of Chronic Facial Pain and Obstructive Sleep Apnea," *Current Opinion in Pulmonary Medicine* 22, no. 6 (November 2016): 570-5.

and not warming, moistening, and filtering the air they breathe, patients can get recurrent ear infections that require treatment. While it's crucial to treat the ear infections, it's even more important to determine the cause, which is often found to be mouth breathing. An article in the *American Journal of Orthodontics and Dentofacial Orthopedics* discusses the importance of identifying mouth breathing since it causes malocclusion, and yet many orthodontists struggle to accurately identify a problem with mouth breathing.[44] We need better education on this subject, and it's great to see the specialists recognizing this need.

Lower IQ and behavioral issues. A study conducted in Europe looking at thousands of children found that those who snore actually have a lower IQ as a result of the sleep deprivation, which disrupts their memory consolidation and ability to learn. Memory consolidation is the brain's retaining and filing of all the facts and activities encountered throughout the day for access in the future. That occurs during the deeper stages of sleep.

The quality of sleep plays a crucial role in a child's ability to focus throughout the day. Often, adults point to behavioral issues in children, even to the point of identifying their problems as ADHD. However, often it's just that the child is lacking proper sleep, as Dr. Loghmanee often discusses.

---

44 Julia Garcia Costa, et al., Clinical recognition of mouth breathers by orthodontists: A preliminary study," American *Journal of Orthodontics and Dentofacial Orthopedics*, vol. 152, issue 5 (November 2017): _ Vol 152 _ Issue 5: 646–653.

The "scorecard" for pediatric sleep apnea is an apnea hypopnea index (AHI) of:

- 1-5 = mild

- 5-10 = moderate

- >10 = severe

What's great about identifying these problems at a young age is that they're very treatable and can really change the landscape of the patient's life moving forward. Most parents would do anything for their children that will benefit them indefinitely. Treating TMD and OSA begins with understanding the situation, getting the right diagnosis, and then coming up with a clear-cut treatment plan for the child. Remember: diagnosis is 95 percent of effective treatment.

SEAN'S VICTORY

Sean was suffering from many of the aforementioned symptoms. While he was a very pleasant young boy, in his earliest visits he did not sit still in the chair. He would try to hang from the dental light, pretending it was a spaceship. It was tough to get him to cooperate, but nonetheless, we at least understood the reason for this behavior after we got the results of his sleep test.

Sean needed a greater ability to breathe through his nose and adequate room for his tongue. By expanding his maxilla, we increased his nasal volume, which also allowed his tongue to rest high in his palate. That helped push his maxilla forward, opening his airway from both a lateral (side-to-side) and an anterior-posterior (front-to-back) dimension. We were also able to help facilitate forward growth of his mandible, which allowed more space for his tongue and further improved his airway volume. This was all quantifiable through CBCT technology and close observation as we monitored his progress.

Throughout treatment, we also discussed dietary and other changes with his mom that could help Sean progress further.

We delivered his upper and lower expanders in February and started activating his appliances to initiate his orthopedic development. In his monthly follow-up visits, his mom began reporting improvements: his snoring was beginning to resolve, his behavior at school was getting better, and his agitation improved immensely.

In fact, in June, Sean showed us how much his grades and school performance had improved by sharing with us his report card—straight A's!

Come September, expansion was complete, and we were ready to do a follow-up validation sleep study to confirm that we had controlled his apneic events and had established proper nasal breathing and improved facial development. The results of his validation sleep study were nothing short of amazing. During that night of sleep, he only had one event in which his breathing slowed enough to wake him up. His oxygen levels maintained at a healthy level throughout the night, his AHI was within normal limits, and his OSA was satisfactorily resolved.

At the end of treatment, Sean was doing very well: His cognitive function, behavior, and sleep had improved dramatically. When he came for a visit, he sat still in the chair and was a very well-behaved patient. The changes that we saw in him were simply astounding—his problems had all been caused by his inability to breathe adequately while he was sleeping at night. Thankfully, he was able to discontinue the use of his medications, since we had found and treated the source of his problems.

Moving forward, we must ensure that proper facial development continues. To do that, we'll maintain Sean's nasal patency (the openness of his nose), helping him to continue breathing adequately through his nose so that he grows and develops to his full genetic potential. We will continue to monitor Sean yearly and coordinate with his orthodontist on how to proceed with his orthodontic treatment in the future, if it is needed. Our goal is to avoid having his apnea return, and we can do our best to ensure this by monitoring his facial development, inquiring about his sleep, and watching his social behavior and how he's performing in school.

Often, with pediatric patients, I'm asked by patients and other providers how we know we've done enough. Dr. Christian Guilleminault eloquently states: "Elimination of oral breathing, i.e., restoration of nasal breathing during wake and sleep, may be the only valid end point when treating OSA. Preventive measures in at-risk groups, such as premature infants, and usage of myofunctional therapy as part of the treatment of OSA are proposed to be important approaches to treat appropriately SBD and its multiple co-morbidities."[45] It is this thought process that needs to be taught to all providers of pediatric patients, because Dr. Guilleminault's research shows that 75 percent of children treated with tonsil and adenoidectomy relapse after four years.[46] That is exactly what happened to Sean.

So the utopia for children is to achieve proper functional nasal breathing where the tongue is in the ideal position, resting high in the palate, to ensure that they have proper facial development moving forward.

In the next chapter, I'll discuss some of the treatment modalities, team members, and features of the TMJ & Sleep Therapy Centre of Northern Indiana that elevate us and make us a unique resource for many patients.

---

45   Christian Guilleminault and Shannon S. Sullivan, "Towards Restoration of Continuous Nasal Breathing as an Alternate Treatment Goal in Pediatric Obstructive Sleep Apnea," *Enliven Archive* 1, no. 1 (2014): 1–5.

46   Ibid.

CHAPTER 10
WHAT ELEVATES OUR TEAM

Great treatment requires a great
team ... we are here for you!

What elevates us at the TMJ & Sleep Therapy Centre of Northern Indiana is our drive to never give up. With every patient, we commit to doing everything we can to uncover the root cause of their problem and improve their quality of life. I pride myself on not stopping until we get to the bottom of the problem and you get the results you're looking for. If I don't have all the answers, I will search for someone who does.

Let me share with you Brittney's story as an example of what I mean. At age thirty-three, Brittney came to see us for help in relieving her pain in her ears, eyes, and face along with dizziness and Meniere's disease, a chronic condition of the inner ear that causes vertigo, progressive hearing loss, and ringing in the ears. At the time, she was taking seven medications for her Meniere's disease and migraines, and she had undergone multiple treatments for both conditions, but nothing had been done to address her TMD.

As a child, she'd had her adenoids and tonsils removed, and she'd even undergone a sleep study in the past, but no significant improvements were ever made. Basically, she was in management mode and was told that her pain and Meniere's were conditions she would have to live with the rest of her life.

Fortunately, she found us via a Google search and came in for an evaluation, driving an hour and a half to see if we might be able to help.

Brittney's victory was to get relief from her headaches, dizziness, and eye and facial pain.

—— VICTORY ——

Brittney's victory was to get relief from her headaches, dizziness, and eye and facial pain.

During her comprehensive evaluation, we found significant inflammation inside Brittney's TM joints, and we explained to her the correlation between TMD, dizziness, and referred ear pain. Her diagnosis was capsulitis of the TM joints and mouth breathing. She had a great deal of inflammation inside the TM joints, causing significant discomfort, and her perpetual mouth breathing was contributing to that disease process. Happily, we were certain that we'd be able to help initiate treatment and begin to get her on a path of significant relief based on the problems we were able to diagnose.

A SPIRIT OF COMFORT

At the TMJ & Sleep Therapy Centre of Northern Indiana, we try to embody a spirit of comfort. We want patients to feel welcome, at home, and important from the moment they walk into our office. We spend a lot of time getting to know patients; we're there to listen to your concerns, to ensure that all your questions are answered, and to determine whether we can, in fact, help you. If for some reason I feel that we cannot help you with your chief complaints and what you're searching for, again, we'll do our very best to get you in touch with the best practitioner we feel might be suitable for you.

We are not just another office that dabbles in treating patients with pain and sleep problems. I have dedicated my life and career to treating these disorders. I am currently the only doctor within a hundred-mile radius of South Bend, Indiana, that is triple-board certified in craniofacial pain and dental sleep medicine. It is now my life's work.

We have a unique team of multidiscipline providers specifically trained to help patients with craniofacial pain and sleep breathing problems.

I think you'll enjoy our welcoming office culture; we get compliments from patients daily about how much they like coming to our office because of our great team. My team is my greatest strength and I am very grateful for their commitment to me and, more importantly, their commitment to you.

COMPREHENSIVE DIAGNOSTICS

One of the hallmark benefits of being a patient of ours is that we have comprehensive diagnostics all under one roof. If you are a candidate for a comprehensive evaluation, you will leave with results of these diagnostic tests on the day of your visit and have a clear-cut treatment plan.

Some of the technologies that allow us to conduct those tests include:

- **Cone beam computed tomography (CBCT)**. It's no secret that the more anatomical information available, the better we are able to diagnose and plan. The CBCT is an on-site, 3-D X-ray unit that captures information not possible with 2-D X-rays. It captures that data using an incredibly low dose of radiation, which puts the patient at minimal risk—something we take very seriously. In fact, the X-rays we take using the CBCT are about equal to the radiation a person gets just from living on Earth in a day's time.

- **Joint vibration analysis (JVA)** measures the friction inside the TM joint. Simple sensors are placed in front of the ears, and the patient is instructed to open and close their mouth so that the vibrations can be recorded. Human joints have surfaces that rub together as they function. Smooth, well-lubricated surfaces and proper biomechanical relationships produce little friction and little vibration, but surface changes such as those caused by degeneration, tears, or displacement of discs generally produce friction and vibration.

  Different disorders can produce different vibration patterns and signatures. We use this technology to accurately diagnose your specific condition. It is a painless, fast, and accurate test. Results are reviewed at the appointment, and the results are part of the diagnostic plan.

- **Cold laser therapy**, commonly referred to as photobiomodulation therapy (PBMT), laser therapy, and low-level laser therapy, is a therapeutic laser modality. We use the Multiwave Locked System (MLS), the most advanced laser therapy on the market. Reduced response times—and overall treatment times—distinguish the MLS laser therapy from traditional laser therapy, with reciprocal advantages for both the operator and the patient. I am able to quickly adapt this technology and see improvements in the patient's quality of life, including, most notably, reduction in pain and swelling and an increase in mobility.

MLS technology delivers therapeutic wavelengths at 808 nanometers, which is anti-endemic and anti-inflammatory, and 905 nanometers, which is an analgesic, allowing tissue penetration of about three to four centimeters. An energetic synergy is created when delivering these wavelengths, and it produces greater anti-inflammatory and analgesic effects than any other can produce on its own, while minimizing the risk of thermal damage to the tissue. It's this unique combination and synchronization of continuous and pulsed emissions that characterizes the MLS and distinguishes it from other lasers.

While this laser has high levels of efficacy, it is extremely safe and provides consistency in treatment. Current literature supports the benefits of PBMT, and some recent studies show as high as a 50 percent decrease in pain upon the first treatment.

- **MediByte** is a diagnostic home sleep test system with straps that attach to the chest and stomach. The beauty of the equipment is that it gathers extremely accurate data while allowing the patient to do a one-night sleep study in the confines of their own home. While only a board-certified sleep physician can diagnose the presence of OSA, MediByte allows us to administer the sleep test through our office and send the results to our colleagues and practitioners to help get the proper diagnosis. We have multiple MediByte units in our office and use them on a daily basis with our patients at the beginning and end of treatment.

While we offer comprehensive diagnostics and care in our office, given the complexity of the health care problems we tackle, we also collaborate with other medical and dental colleagues for collaboration and help in treating patients. Some of the medical specialists we routinely partner with include physicians specializing in ENT, sleep, osteopathic medicine, primary care, rheumatology, neurology, pulmonology, pain management, chiropractic, physical medicine and rehabilitation, and pediatrics. We also have great relationships with physical therapists, speech pathologists, mental health therapists, nutritionists, dietitians, and wellness coaches.

We find that using a team approach and collaborating with other health care providers delivers the best results for our patients. If your treatment plan includes help from another practitioner, we will get you in touch with them, help coordinate your appointments, and ensure they have all the diagnostic information needed to collaborate with us about your care.

Your treatment will be a customized plan that's specific to you—and only you. We do not have a cookie-cutter approach to care, and everyone's treatment plan is distinctly different. Again, compliance is a great determinant of treatment success. As my father taught me, we can only help a patient as much as they're willing to help themselves. Your success is important to us, and I can guarantee that we will be with you every step of the way. But if you want a victory, you have to commit to the process. We can't achieve the best results without you taking an active role in your own treatment, and we are here to help you each step along the way.

Brittney did just that, and the results speak for themselves.

BRITTNEY'S VICTORY

We began Brittney's treatment in April. She was compliant with all of our home-care recommendations and lifestyle changes, in addition to the orthotics we fabricated to treat her TMD. Within twelve weeks of starting treatment, Brittney reported that her dizziness, eye pain, and maxilla and mandible pain were completely gone, and her facial and headache pain were nearly gone. At twelve weeks, we began weaning Brittney off her orthotics, and she was able to resume normal use of her maxilla and mandible without her daytime orthotic in place. At that point in her treatment, she also reported that all of her pain was completely gone—100 percent resolved within twelve weeks.

Since she no longer had symptoms of Meniere's disease, she wanted to know if the problem all along was TMD. We recommended that she follow up with an ENT physician to see if the diagnosis of Meniere's disease could be eliminated from her medical history, since she was now asymptomatic for the first time. In the end, the Meniere's diagnosis no longer mattered to Brittney; what mattered to her was that her pain and dizziness were gone and that the root of her problems had been discovered. That's what ultimately resolved her problems.

The most touching part of Brittney's treatment was when she offered to do a video testimonial for us. When asked "How has treatment helped you?" Brittney replied through tears, "The best part … is to be alive again."

It's a privilege and an honor for me and my staff to help patients like Brittney and the others shared in this book get their lives back again.

Here's what a few other patients have said about the TMJ & Sleep Therapy Centre of Northern Indiana.:

I woke up in pain every day with my jaw clenched tightly. I began having pain in my neck, shoulders, and lower back. I started having problems with my teeth/jaw lining up when I would close my mouth. The treatment helped me greatly reduce my pain, controlling my clenching and realigning my jaw into a natural, comfortable position. I couldn't believe how quickly the staff knew me by name! Each time I came, I was greeted by the friendly staff who made it obvious they truly care about their patients! They were also helpful when it came to helping me navigate the insurance process. ~ Rachel H.

My general practitioner thought I was having a stroke as I was having ear pain, and facial numbness on the left side. There was so much pain I couldn't do anything. Now I can function and take care of my obligations and graduate school. ~ Michele T.

I would stop breathing at night and gasp for air. My husband said my snore was pretty loud too. I feel more rested in the morning, my jaw doesn't hurt, I sleep more soundly. (The staff) are so nice and answer all my questions. Best staff around. —Nancy H.

ORTHOTICS AND ORAL APPLIANCES

... WHAT DO THEY LOOK LIKE?

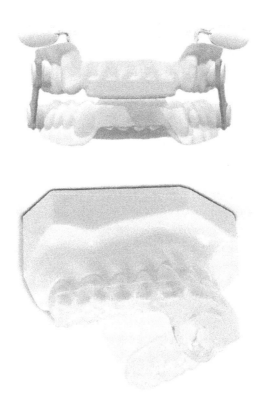

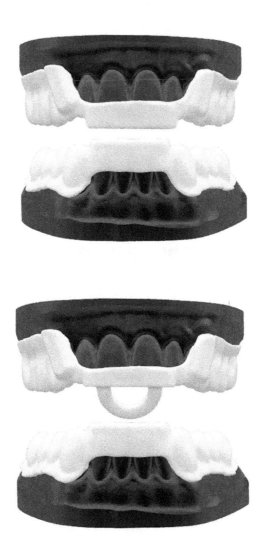

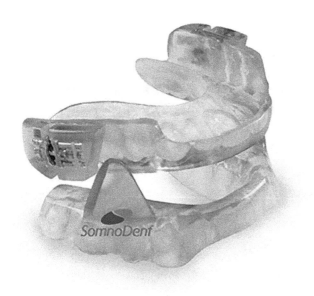

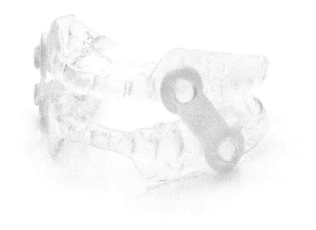

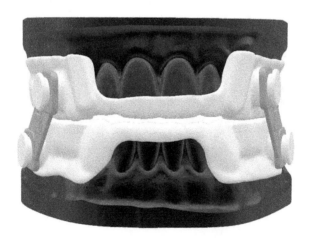

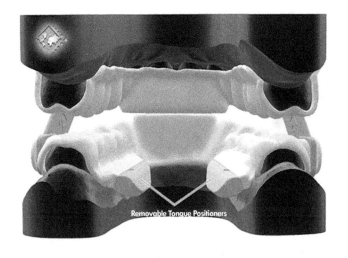

Removable Tongue Positioners

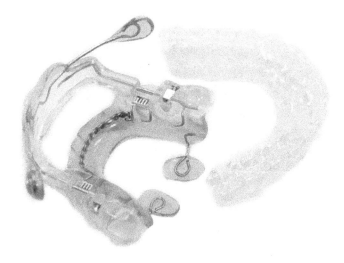

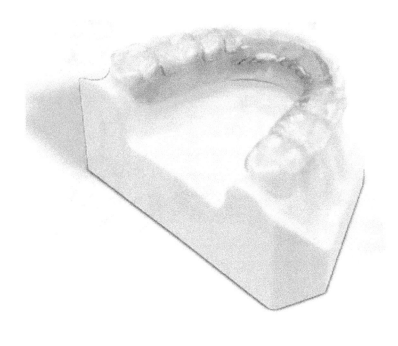

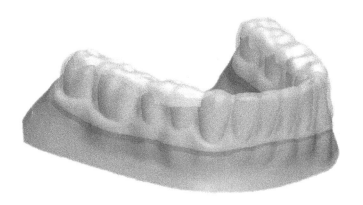

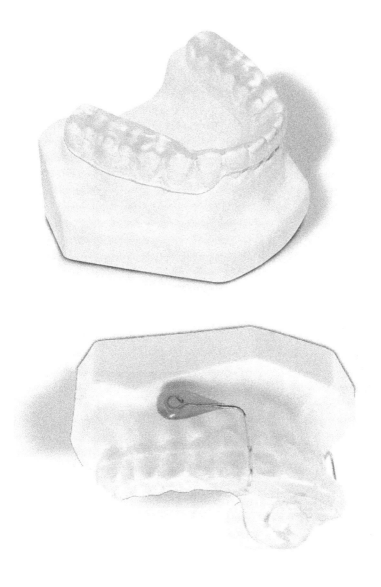

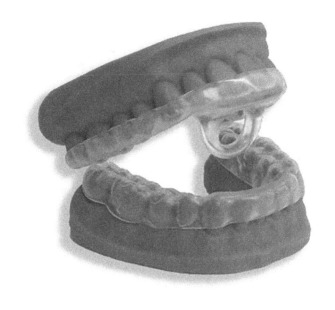

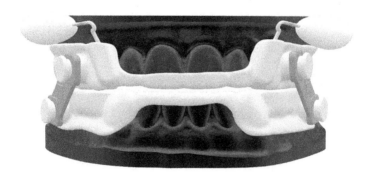

CONCLUSION
ENVISION A LIFE
WITHOUT PAIN

What would a victory look like to you? So many patients have completely forgotten what it's like to be "normal." People get accustomed to feeling groggy in the mornings, hitting the snooze button multiple times, waking with a headache and reaching for a pain med. They don't even remember what it's like to just rise out of bed in the morning and have energy and go on about their day with no dizzy spells, no vision problems, no chewing problems, and pain-free.

A lot of people have been told by various health care providers that they can't get better, and they will have to live with their pain for the rest of their life. They've been told that the way they are living now is their norm.

Your norm today doesn't have to be your norm tomorrow. Every day, we see patients who are ultimately able to turn their lives around. We are able to help them recreate normal. That means getting out of bed refreshed, going through the day upright and awake and without pain, and leading a life filled with energy that lets them take on the day.

At the TMJ & Sleep Therapy Centre of Northern Indiana, we give patients hope. We "give them permission" to fight their pain and get better. Sometimes that's all it takes for a patient to begin to turn things around. They just need someone to tell them that getting rid of their chronic pain is doable.

It's absolutely worth taking a little time to investigate the treatments at the TMJ & Sleep Therapy Centre of Northern Indiana. You may find that there is a solution to your pain, a solution that can turn your life around. We only initiate treatment if we truly believe we can help you. Above all, we want to give you answers, we want to help you figure out the source of your pain—that's the way to get better, whether we provide the treatment or we find a referral provider to help.

As you can surely tell, I take my expertise and life-changing approach of a person's health very seriously. I also take you, your comfort, and your confidence in what's next very personally. Because I know that pain can zap the joy from your life. But you don't have to live with it. You can take control of your health, you can *be the victor over TMD and sleep apnea.*

TMJ & Sleep Therapy Centre
1245 East University Drive
Granger, IN 46530
Phone: (574) 968-5166
info@tmjsleepindiana.com
https://www.tmjsleepindiana.com/

HOW IMPORTANT IS A VICTORY TO YOU?

If you are having symptoms of TMD and/or OSA, chances are you're having trouble getting answers. Take these quick quizzes to see if it's time for you to schedule a visit with us at the TMJ & Sleep Therapy Centre of Northern Indiana.

PAIN QUIZ

Do you take over-the-counter or prescription medication more than once a week for head or face pain?
Yes ___ No ___

Do you wake with headaches in the morning?
Yes ___ No ___

Does your jaw or face often feel sore or tired?

Yes ___ No ___

Do you have clicking or popping or noises in your jaw joint?

Yes ___ No ___

Is your jaw opening limited or asymmetrical?

Yes ___ No ___

Does stress aggravate or create head or face pain?

Yes ___ No ___

Does your pain limit your ability to do daily activities?

Yes ___ No ___

*If you answered yes to any of the questions above,
you may be at risk of TMD.*

SLEEP QUIZ

Do you snore loudly?

Yes ___ No ___

Do you often feel tired or fatigued after sleep?

Yes ___ No ___

Has anyone noticed that you quit breathing during sleep?

Yes ___ No ___

Do you take medication for high blood pressure?
Yes ____ No ____

Have you recently dozed off watching TV?
Yes ____ No ____

Have you recently dozed off sitting inactive in a public place (e.g. a theatre or a meeting)?
Yes ____ No ____

Have you recently dozed off sitting and talking to someone?
Yes ____ No ____

Have you recently dozed off in a car while stopped for a few minutes in traffic?
Yes ____ No ____

If you answered yes to any of the questions above, you may be at risk for OSA.

DEAR PRACTICING DENTISTS,

Now that you are aware of the effects of untreated obstructive sleep apnea and what a life filled with chronic pain looks like, a VICTORY for you may be successfully implementing or growing these services in your practice.

Some find the business operations and marketing of these services to be a challenge and are at a loss of how to implement them. In fact, it was many phones calls, requests to shadow, and inquiries to see how Dr. Klauer operates that led him to work with practices across North America. It was this demand that created the need for Dr. Klauer and his team to offer training and support to help practices achieve their goals. They work with practices of all sizes and in any sized market to help improve their ability to treat patients with pain and sleep problems. Whether you are wanting to improve your current process or are starting a new sleep and pain practice, Dr. Klauer has made it his mission to help every provider offer a world class patient experience.

If You Want to Help More Patients Through Sleep (and Pain) Dentistry, Dr. Klauer Has a Special Gift for You!

As you can tell from this powerful and informative book, Dr. Klauer has mastered all aspects of treating patients' obstructive sleep apnea and helping patients rid their lives of chronic pain.

Every smart Dentist knows it takes more than clinical knowhow to be able to truly help patients. You must have sound and effective business systems to educate and serve your patients in the most professional way possible.

To learn about this proven system that Dr. Klauer and his world class team have created—which now helps save, change and improve the lives of thousands of patients a year (a number constantly growing)—you can request your own copy of his Ultimate Sleep Success System Fast Start Program that he has generously decided to gift to every dentist who reads this book.

You can find all the details at
www.SleepSuccessSystem.com

Get Your Copy of Dr. Klauer's Sleep Success Book for Dentists at **www.SleepSuccessSystem.com**

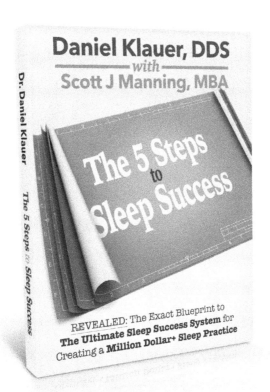

CPSIA information can be obtained
at www.ICGtesting.com
Printed in the USA
LVHW04s1953031018
592294LV00012B/28/P